Acknowledgements

This report was prepared by the Department of Health and Human Services in collaboration with the Department of Education and the Department of Justice. It is an outgrowth of the *Surgeon General's Report on Mental Health* which was released in December, 1999.

Interdepartmental Planning Committee

Co-chairs

Beverly L. Malone, Ph.D, RN, FAAN
Deputy Assistant Secretary for Health
Office of Public Health and Science

Kimberly Hoagwood, Ph.D.
Associate Director for Child and
 Adolescent Research
National Institute of Mental Health

Coordinating Editor
S. Serene Olin, Ph.D.

Members

Coleen Boyle, Ph.D.
Terry Cline, Ph.D.
Marsha Davenport, M.D.
Connie Deshpande, B.A., M.P.A.
Margaret Feerick, Ph.D.
Jerry Flanzer, D.S.W.
Norma Hatot, Capt, USPHS
Lynne Haverkos, M.D., M.P.H.
Kelly Henderson, Ph.D.
Judith Katz-Leavy, M.Ed.
Woodie S. Kessel, M.D., M.P.H.
Catherine A. Lesesne, M.P.H.

Peggy McCardle, Ph.D., M.P.H.
Suzanne Martone, M.P.A.
Martha Moorehouse, Ph.D.
Eve Moscicki, Sc.D., M.P.H.
Dianne Murphy, M.D.
Allan S. Noonan, M.D., M.P.H.
Delores Parron, Ph.D.
William Rodriguez, M.D.
Rolando Santiago, Ph.D.
Karen Stern, Ph.D.
Frank Sullivan, M.D.
John J. Tuskan, Jr., R.N., M.S.N.

Other Contributors

Betty James
Damon Thompson
Marilyn Weeks

Clarissa Wittenberg
Daisy Whittemore
Catherine West

Substantial public input was sought and received at multiple steps in the process of developing the action agenda for children's mental health. Special thanks to all who contributed to the national dialogue on children's mental health, especially to:
• All who provided input through the World Wide Web and the mail;
• Participants at the Surgeon General's Listening Session; and
• Participants at the Surgeon General's Conference on Children's Mental Health, especially the youth whose input reminded us of the critical need to listen to their perspectives.

Special thanks to the leadership and staff of the Office of Public Health and Science for their enthusiastic support of this interdepartmental effort.
Nicole Lurie, M.D., M.S.P.H., *Principal Deputy Assistant Secretary for Health*
Kenneth Moritsugu, M.D., M.P.H., *Deputy Surgeon General, USPHS*

Suggested Citation:
U.S. Public Health Service, Report of the Surgeon General 's Conference on Children's Mental Health:
A National Action Agenda. Was hington, DC: Department of Health and Human Services, 2000

Surgeon General's Conference on

Children's Mental Health: Developing a National Action Agenda

September 18-19, 2000

Sponsored by

DEPARTMENT OF HEALTH AND HUMAN SERVICES

Office of the Surgeon General, Office of Public Health and Science

National Institute of Mental Health, National Institutes of Health

Center for Mental Health Services, Substance Abuse and Mental Health Services Administration

Assistant Secretary for Planning and Evaluation, Office of the Secretary

National Center for Environmental Health, Centers for Disease Control and Prevention

Food and Drug Administration

Maternal and Child Health Bureau, Health Resources and Services Administration

National Institute on Drug Abuse, National Institutes of Health

DEPARTMENT OF EDUCATION

Office of Special Education Programs, Office of Special Education and Rehabilitative Services

DEPARTMENT OF JUSTICE

Office of Juvenile Justice and Delinquency Prevention, Office of Justice Programs

In collaboration with

Office of Safe and Drug-Free Schools, Office of Elementary and Secondary Education, Department of Education

Administration on Children, Youth and Families, Administration for Children and Families, Department of Health and Human Services

Health Care Financing Administration, Department of Health and Human Services

National Institute of Child Health and Human Development, National Institutes of Health, Department of Health and Human Services

Foreword

The burden of suffering experienced by children with mental health needs and their families has created a health crisis in this country. Growing numbers of children are suffering needlessly because their emotional, behavioral, and developmental needs are not being met by those very institutions which were explicitly created to take care of them. It is time that we as a Nation took seriously the task of preventing mental health problems and treating mental illnesses in youth.

The mental health needs of our children have elicited interest from the highest level of government, including the White House and members of both the House of Representatives and the Senate. This *Report of the Surgeon General's Conference on Children's Mental Health*: *A National Action Agenda* represents an extraordinary level of collaboration among three major Federal Departments: the Department of Health and Human Services, the Department of Education, and the Department of Justice.

This report introduces a blueprint for addressing children's mental health in the United States. It reflects the culmination of a number of significant activities over the past year. On March 20, 2000, a White House Meeting launched a new public-private effort to improve the appropriate diagnosis and treatment of children with emotional and behavioral conditions. Serious concerns were raised about the appropriate diagnosis and treatment of emotional and behavioral difficulties in children, and the need to take steps to address this issue. On June 26, 2000, I hosted the Surgeon General's Listening Session on Children's Mental

Health. Input on critical issues in children's mental health was solicited from the public through the World Wide Web and by mailing requests to over 500 individuals. Approximately 50 individuals were invited to provide input at a day of thoughtful discussion about the gaps in our knowledge on children's mental health. This input helped shape the agenda for a national conference.

On September 18 and 19, 2000, the *Surgeon General's Conference on Children's Mental Health: Developing a National Action Agenda* was held in Washington, DC. Three hundred participants were invited, representing a broad cross-section of mental health stakeholders, including youth and family members, professional organizations and associations, advocacy groups, faith-based practitioners, clinicians, educators, healthcare providers, and members of the scientific community and the healthcare industry. This conference enlisted the help of the participants in developing specific recommendations for a National Action Agenda on Children's Mental Health. A related meeting on *Psychopharmacology for Young Children: Clinical Needs and Research Opportunities,* was held by the National Institute of Mental Health and the Food and Drug Administration on October 2nd and 3rd, 2000. Recommendations from these two meetings formed the basis of this national action agenda.

One of the chief priorities in the Office of the Surgeon General and Assistant Secretary for Health has been to work to ensure that every child has an optimal chance for a healthy start in life. When we think about a healthy start, we often limit our

1

focus to physical health. But, as clearly articulated in the Surgeon General's Report on Mental Health, mental health is fundamental to overall health and well-being. And that is why we must ensure that our health system responds as readily to the needs of children's mental health as it does to their physical well-being.

One way to do so is to move the country towards a community health system that balances health promotion, disease prevention, early detection and universal access to care. That system must include a balanced research agenda, including basic, biomedical, clinical, behavioral, health services, school-based and community-based prevention and intervention research, and it must include a new invigorated approach to mental health. There is no mental health equivalent to the federal government's commitment to childhood immunization. Children and families are suffering because of missed opportunities for prevention and early identification, fragmented services, and low priorities for resources. Overriding all of this is the issue of stigma, which continues to surround mental illness.

Mental healthcare is dispersed across multiple systems: schools, primary care, the juvenile justice system, child welfare and substance abuse treatment. But the first system is the family, and this agenda reflects the voices of youth and family. The vision and goals outlined in this agenda represent an unparalleled opportunity to make a difference in the quality of life for America's children.

David Satcher, M.D., Ph.D.
Assistant Secretary for Health and Surgeon General

Overarching Vision

Mental health is a critical component of children's learning and general health. Fostering social and emotional health in children as a part of healthy child development must therefore be a national priority. Both the promotion of mental health in children and the treatment of mental disorders should be major public health goals. To achieve these goals, the Surgeon General's National Action Agenda for Children's Mental Health takes as its guiding principles a commitment to:

1) Promoting the recognition of mental health as an essential part of child health;
2) Integrating family, child and youth-centered mental health services into all systems that serve children and youth;
3) Engaging families and incorporating the perspectives of children and youth, in the development of all mental healthcare planning;
4) Developing and enhancing a public-private health infrastructure to support these efforts to the fullest extent possible.

Goals

1. Promote public awareness of children's mental health issues and reduce stigma associated with mental illness.

2. Continue to develop, disseminate, and implement scientifically-proven prevention and treatment services in the field of children's mental health.

3. Improve the assessment and recognition of mental health needs in children.

4. Eliminate racial/ethnic and socioeconomic disparities in access to mental healthcare.

5. Improve the infrastructure for children's mental health services including support for scientifically-proven interventions across professions.

6. Increase access to and coordination of quality mental healthcare services.

7. Train frontline providers to recognize and manage mental health issues, and educate mental health providers in scientifically-proven prevention and treatment services.

8. Monitor the access to and coordination of quality mental healthcare services.

Goal 1: Promote public awareness of children's mental health issues and reduce stigma associated with mental illness.

ACTION STEPS

➤ Promote social, emotional, and behavioral well-being as an integral part of a child's health development.

➤ Develop and/or disseminate existing guidelines on how to enhance child development, including mental health. Different sets of guidelines will need to be created for the general public, families, parents and caregivers, and professional groups.

➤ Identify early indicators for mental health problems.

➤ Integrate mental health consultations as part of children's overall general healthcare and advise healthcare providers regarding the importance of assessing for mental health needs.

➤ Develop national capacity to provide adequate preventive mental health services.

➤ Conduct a public education campaign to address the stigma associated with mental health disorders. This could be accomplished through partnerships with the media, youth, public health systems, communities, health professionals, and advocacy groups.

Goal 2: Continue to develop, disseminate, and implement scientifically-proven prevention and treatment services in the field of children's mental health.

ACTION STEPS

➢ Support basic research on child development, and the use of knowledge about neurological, cognitive, social, and psychological development to design better screening, assessment, and treatment tools and to develop prevention efforts.

➢ Support research on familial, cultural, and ecological contexts to identify opportunities for promoting mental health in children and providing effective prevention, treatment, and services.

➢ Support research in developmental psychopathology to help clarify diagnoses and provide methodology that is sensitive, specific, and that can be used in designing and interpreting pharmacological and other clinical trials.

➢ Support research in basic and clinical neuroscience to provide better information and understanding of pharmacogenetics and ontogeny of drug effects on the developing brain in the short term, as well as the long-term consequences of pharmacological intervention, associated with both acute and chronic exposure.

➢ Support research on legal/ethical and confidentiality issues associated with the treatment of children and families.

➢ Support research to develop and test innovative behavioral, pharmacological, and multimodal interventions.

➢ Increase research on proven treatments, practices, and services developed in the laboratory to assess their effectiveness in real-world settings.

➢ Study the nature and effectiveness of clinical practices in real-world settings.

➢ Assess the short- and long-term outcomes of prevention and treatment efforts, including the effect of early intervention on prognosis and course of mental illness.

➢ Promote research on factors that facilitate or impede the implementation and dissemination of scientifically-proven interventions.

➢ Support research evaluating the process and impact of promising policies and programs, including cost-effectiveness research (e.g., EPSDT, IDEA, Head Start, SCHIP [see Appendix B]).

➢ Evaluate the impact of organization and financing of services on access, the use of scientifically-proven prevention and treatment services, and outcomes for children and families.

➢ Develop and evaluate model programs that can be disseminated and sustained in the community.

➢ Build private and public partnerships to facilitate the dissemination and cross-fertilization of knowledge.

➢ Create a forum for promoting direct communication among researchers, providers, youth and families to bridge the gap between research and practice.

➢ Create a standing workgroup for the purpose of identifying research opportunities, discussing potential approaches, monitoring progress in the area of psychopharmacology for young children, and addressing ethical issues regarding research with children. This group should include representatives of all interested parties, such as researchers, practitioners, youth and families, industry, and federal regulatory, research, and services agencies.

➤ Create an oversight system to identify and approve scientifically-based prevention and treatment interventions, promote their use, and monitor their implementation.

Goal 3: Improve the assessment and recognition of mental health needs in children.

ACTION STEPS

➤ Encourage early identification of mental health needs in existing preschool, childcare, education, health, welfare, juvenile justice, and substance abuse treatment systems.

➤ Create tangible tools for practitioners in these systems to help them assess children's social and emotional needs, discuss mental health issues with parents/caregivers and children, and make appropriate referrals for further assessments or interventions.

➤ Train all primary healthcare providers and educational personnel in ways to enhance child mental health and recognize early indicators of mental health problems, including among children with special health care needs, children of fragmented families, and children of parents with mental health and/or substance abuse disorders.

➤ Promote cost-effective, proactive systems of behavior support at the school level. These systems of behavior support should emphasize universal, primary prevention methods that recognize the unique differences of all children and

youth, but include selective individual student supports for those who have more intense and long-term needs.

➤ Increase provider understanding and training to address the various mental health issues among children with special health care needs and their families.

➤ Increase the understanding of practitioners, policymakers, and the public of the role that untreated mental health problems play in placing children and youth at risk for entering the juvenile justice system.

Goal 4: Eliminate racial/ethnic and socioeconomic disparities in access to mental healthcare.

ACTION STEPS

➤ Increase accessible, culturally competent, scientifically-proven services that are sensitive to youth and family strengths and needs.

➤ Increase efforts to recruit and train minority providers who represent the racial, ethnic, and cultural diversity of the country.

➤ Co-locate mental health services with other key systems (e.g., education, primary care, welfare, juvenile justice, substance abuse treatment) to improve access, especially in remote or rural communities.

➤ Strengthen the resource capacity of schools to serve as a key link to a comprehensive, seamless system of school- and community-based identification, assessment and treatment services, to meet the needs of youth and their families where they are.

➤ Encourage the development and integration of alternative, testable approaches to engage families in prevention and intervention strategies (e.g., pastoral counseling).

➤ Develop policies for uninsured children across diverse populations and geographic areas to address the problem of disparities in mental health access.

➤ Develop and support mental health programs designed to divert youth with mental health problems from the juvenile justice system.

➤ Increase research on diagnosis, prevention, treatment, and service delivery to address disparities, especially among different racial, ethnic, gender, sexual orientation, and socioeconomic groups.

Goal 5: Improve the infrastructure for children's mental health services including support for scientifically-proven interventions across professions.

ACTION STEPS

➤ Encourage the health system to respond to mental health prevention and treatment service needs through universal, comprehensive, and continuous health coverage.

➤ Review both incentives and disincentives for healthcare providers to assess the mental health needs of children, including preventive interventions, screening, and referral.

➤ Provide the infrastructure for cost-effective, cross-system collaboration and integrated care, including support to healthcare providers for

identification, treatment coordination, and/or referral to specialty services; and the development of integrated community networks to increase appropriate referral opportunities.

➤ Provide incentives for scientifically-proven and cost-effective prevention and treatment interventions that are organized to support families, and that consider children and their caregivers as a basic unit (e.g., family therapy, home-based treatment, intensive case management).

➤ Create incentives and support for agencies, programs and individual practitioners to develop and utilize science-based strategies and interventions in community settings.

➤ Determine which policies and programs for children are most cost-effective and improve access to quality care, especially among the uninsured.

Goal 6: Increase access to and coordination of quality mental healthcare services.

ACTION STEPS

➤ Develop a common language to describe children's mental health, emphasizing adaptive functioning and taking into account ecological, cultural and familial context. A common language is important to facilitate service delivery across systems.

➤ Develop a universal measurement system across all major service sectors that is age-appropriate, culturally-competent, and gender sensitive to (i) identify children, including those with special health care needs, who may need mental health services; (ii) track child progress during treatment; and (iii) measure treatment outcomes for individual patients.

➤ Modify definitions and evaluation procedures used by education systems to identify and serve children and youth who have mental health needs. These definitions and procedures should facilitate access to, not exclusion from, essential services.

➤ Provide access to services in places where youth and families congregate (e.g., schools, recreation centers, churches, and others).

➤ Support the development of coordinated responses by emergency medical providers (e.g., paramedics, emergency room personnel) and community mental health service providers to expedite appropriate treatment and/or referral for children presenting with emergency and traumatic episodes in hospital emergency rooms.

➤ Address issues of confidentiality in ways that respect a family's right to privacy, but encourage coordination and collaboration among providers in different systems.

➤ Encourage family organizations to help family members access information on how to enhance children's mental health and effective treatments for mental illness so that they can make fully-informed decisions about interventions offered.

➤ Include youth in treatment planning by offering them direct information in developmentally appropriate ways about service options. As much as possible, allow youth to make decisions and choices about preferred intervention strategies.

➤ Use family advocates, such as family members with prior experience, to assist families in interacting effectively with complicated service

systems such as healthcare, education, juvenile justice, child welfare, and substance abuse treatment.

➤ Provide a mechanism for input from youth and families in setting a national mental health agenda and in assessing policies and programs to promote mental health services delivery.

Goal 7: Train frontline providers to recognize and manage mental health issues, and educate mental health providers in scientifically-proven prevention and treatment services.

ACTION STEPS

➤ Engage professional organizations in educating new frontline providers in various systems (e.g. teachers, physicians, nurses, hospital emergency personnel, daycare providers, probation officers, and other child healthcare providers) in child development; equip them with skills to address and enhance children's mental health; and train them to recognize early symptoms of emotional or behavioral problems for proactive intervention. Such training must focus on developmental and cultural differences in cognitive, social, emotional, and behavioral functioning, and understanding these issues in familial and ecological context.

➤ Facilitate training of new providers by building knowledge of child development into the existing curricula of professional programs and encouraging on-going training opportunities across disciplines to facilitate the development of effective partnerships.

➤ Develop and evaluate multidisciplinary programs for healthcare professionals that focus on child and family mental health.

➤ Create training support for professionals, paraprofessionals, and family advocates to keep abreast of new developments in the field of children's mental health.

➤ Address the shortage of well-trained child mental health specialists, particularly minority individuals, through active recruitment and incentive efforts by professional organizations, federal programs, and federal legislation, and consider the development of training programs for mid-level providers in mental health to address inadequate capacity.

➤ Engage professional boards for mental health specialists (e.g., psychiatry, psychology, social work, and nursing) to require training in: evidence-based prevention and treatment interventions; outcome-based quality assurance; competency-based assessment and diagnostic skills; principles of culturally-competent care; and engaging youth and families as partners in assessment, intervention, and outcome monitoring.

➤ Ensure mechanisms to monitor and evaluate efforts to train new professionals, retrain existing professionals, and examine the effectiveness of these training efforts.

Goal 8: Monitor the access to and coordination of quality mental healthcare services.

ACTION STEPS

➤ Establish formal partnerships among federal research, regulatory, and service agencies, professional associations and families/caregivers to facilitate the transfer of knowledge among research, practice, and policy related to children's mental health.

➤ Encourage behavioral healthcare industry and service agencies to develop and use broad-based outcome and process measures to ensure accountability. These measures should be relevant and meaningful, such as symptom severity, adaptive functioning, family satisfaction, and societal costs and benefits in terms of involvement in systems such as special education, welfare, and juvenile justice.

➤ Develop national quality improvement protocols that emphasize the use of scientifically-proven practices and evaluate the effectiveness of service systems.

➤ Encourage providers to inform consumers about evidence for and against the effectiveness of proposed treatments and services.

➤ Make available information on effective prevention and treatment interventions through federal partners, professional organizations, family organizations, and private foundations. In addition, provide information that will allow practitioners to evaluate the worth of promising interventions.

➤ Encourage industry and service agencies to develop a variety of mechanisms for consumers to communicate their experiences and concerns to funding agencies and purchasers of healthcare plans (i.e., federal, state and local governments, and private employers).

➤ Monitor efforts to coordinate services and reduce mental health access disparities through public health surveillance and evaluation research.

Proceedings based on the Surgeon General's Conference on Children's Mental Health:

Developing a National Action Agenda

Conference Summary

Background

The nation is facing a public crisis in mental health for infants, children and adolescents. Many children have mental health problems that interfere with normal development and functioning. In the United States, one in ten children and adolescents suffer from mental illness severe enough to cause some level of impairment. Yet, in any given year, it is estimated that about one in five children receive mental health services. Unmet need for services remains as high now as it was 20 years ago. Recent evidence compiled by the World Health Organization indicates that by the year 2020, childhood neuropsychiatric disorders will rise proportionately by over 50 percent, internationally, to become one of the five most common causes of morbidity, mortality, and disability among children.

Concerns about inappropriate diagnosis—that is, either over- or under-diagnosis—of children's mental health problems and about the availability of evidence-based (i.e., scientifically-proven) treatments and services for children and their families have sparked a national dialogue around these issues. There is broad evidence that the nation lacks a unified infrastructure to help these children and many are falling through the cracks. Too often, children who are not identified as having mental health problems and who do not receive services end up in jail. Children and families are suffering because of missed opportunities for prevention and early identification, fragmented treatment services, and low priorities for resources.

To address these critical issues, the Office of the Surgeon General held a conference on *Children's Mental Health: Developing a National Action Agenda* on September 18 – 19, 2000 in Washington, DC. This conference represented an extraordinary level of collaboration among three major Federal Departments: the Department of Health and Human Services, the Department of Justice, and the Department of Education. The purpose of the conference was to engage a group of thoughtful citizens in a meaningful dialogue about issues involved in prevention, identification, recognition, and referral of children with mental health needs for appropriate, evidence-based treatments or services. The 300 invited presenters and participants represented a broad cross-section of mental health stakeholders, including primary care, education, juvenile justice, child welfare, and substance abuse. Disciplines represented include education, pediatrics, social work, psychiatry, psychology, nursing, public health, and faith-based practitioners. Individuals representing associations, advocacy groups, the scientific community, members of the healthcare industry, clinicians, healthcare providers, families and youth attended this conference.

This conference is one piece of a national conversation addressing the mental health of our Nation's children. The *White House Conference on Mental Health*, in June 1999, was the first major public orientation to the realities of mental illness in the United States. This was followed by the *Surgeon General's Call to Action to Prevent Suicide* in July 1999, and the release of a first-ever *Surgeon*

General's Report on Mental Health in December 1999. This report addressed complex issues in mental health and included a chapter on the mental health of children. Most recently, in March of this year, the White House held another meeting specifically addressing the need to improve the diagnosis and treatment of children with emotional and behavioral conditions. Following this conference, the National Institute of Mental Health and the Food and Drug Administration held a meeting in early October, focusing on research needed to develop psychopharmaceuticals for young children.

The agenda for this meeting was developed with extensive input from a broad range of interested individuals. In May, public input was solicited through the World Wide Web and mailings to over 500 individuals. Nearly 400 responses were received within a month. On June 26, 50 individuals were invited to a formal Listening Session with the Surgeon General to help craft the agenda for this conference. Key issues of concern to families, service providers, and researchers were identified, and included:

■ Educating the public about mental health and illness in children;

■ Ensuring screening and early identification of children within key service systems;

■ Implementing evidence-based treatments and services;

■ Providing adequate and appropriate education and training to frontline providers;

■ Engaging families in all aspects of service delivery; and

■ Continuing to build the research base on children's mental health.

The conference agenda was thus developed to address these major concerns, with the aim of addressing the need to improve the state of children's mental health and their families'. To initiate national dialogue about children's mental health concerns, conference participants listened to plenary sessions in which leaders in the field, including youth and family members themselves, briefly outlined key issues involved in:

■ Identifying, recognizing, and referring children with mental health needs in key services systems;

■ Health services disparities: increasing access to services through family engagement and reducing disparities in access; and

■ State of the evidence in treatments, services, systems of care and financing: the gap between what we know and what we do.

These presentations, summarized below, provided conference participants with information to engage in meaningful discussions on children's mental health issues. Conference participants were divided into 10 working groups over the two days. To help develop consensus recommendations, participants aided by selected facilitators and recorders, were asked to:

■ Identify the barriers to appropriate identification and recognition of children with mental health needs and the factors that impede access to appropriate treatments or services;

■ Identify major opportunities for promoting child and adolescent mental health and for preventing risks and antecedents associated with mental illness;

■ Identify the major policies that offer opportunity for strengthening recognition and improving access to care;

- Identify professional training needs in child and adolescent mental health;

- Identify the major barriers to implementing evidence-based treatments and services; and

- Develop recommendations for bridging the gaps among research, practice, and policy.

Facilitators and recorders of each group helped group members prioritize their recommendations, and came together each day of the conference to synthesize the input from their respective groups. Consensus among the top recommendations was developed, and these were presented to the Surgeon General and the conference participants. Youths present at the conference formed their own group, and presented their input directly to the Surgeon General and the participants as well.

Conference participants also had the opportunity to directly address Dr. Satcher, and to provide their comments. These recommendations, together with those developed from the NIMH/FDA meeting on *Psychopharmacology for Young Children: Clinical Needs and Research Opportunities,* were used as a basis for the development of the Surgeon General's National Action Agenda for Children's Mental Health.

Conference Proceedings

These summary statements reflect the views expressed in the presentations by invited speakers and discussants at the conference.

Welcome
DAVID SATCHER, M.D., Ph.D., Assistant Secretary for Health and Surgeon General

Dr. Satcher applauded the nation's unprecedented focus on children's mental health, and in particular, the interest from the White House and members of both the House of Representatives and the Senate. He shared his struggle with issues of policy and science in his role as both Assistant Secretary for Health and Surgeon General. Dr. Satcher commended the exemplary collaboration among the three Federal Departments: the Department of Health and Human Services, the Department of Education, and the Department of Justice, in this monumental effort. He briefly highlighted the historical context for the development of this conference, including the White House Meeting in March that launched a new public-private effort to improve the appropriate diagnosis and treatment of children with emotional and behavioral conditions; solicitation of public input on children's mental health issues; and the Surgeon General's Listening Session on Children's Mental Health on June 26, 2000. These events helped shaped the agenda for today's conference.

Dr. Satcher said that one of the chief priorities in the Office of the Surgeon General and Assistant Secretary for Health has been to work to ensure that every child has an optimal chance for a healthy start in life. When we think about a healthy start, we often limit our focus to physical health. But, as clearly articulated in the Surgeon General's Report on Mental Health, mental health is fundamental to overall health and well-being. Just as things go wrong with the heart, the lungs, the liver and the kidneys, things go wrong with the brain. And that is why we must ensure that our health system responds as readily to the needs of children's mental health as it does to the needs of their physical well-being.

One way to do so is to move the country towards a community health system that balances health promotion, disease prevention, early detection and offers universal access to care. Such a system must include a balanced research agenda, including basic, biomedical, clinical, behavioral, health services and community-based prevention research, and it must include a new invigorated approach to mental health. Dr. Satcher noted that there is no mental health equivalent to the federal government's commitment to childhood immunization. Children and families are suffering because of missed opportunities for prevention and early identification, fragmented services, and low priorities for resources. Overriding all of this is the issue of stigma, which continues to surround mental illness.

Mental healthcare is dispersed across multiple settings: schools, primary care, the juvenile justice system, and child welfare. But the first system is the family, and the family is represented here today, and probably better represented at this conference than any conference in the history of a Surgeon General's report. To improve services for children with mental health problems and their families, Dr. Satcher stated that we need to take three steps: 1) To improve early recognition and appropriate identification of mental disorders in children within all systems serving children; 2) To improve access to services by removing barriers faced by families with mental health needs, with a specific aim to reduce disparities in access to care; and 3) To close the gap between research and practice, ensuring evidence-based treatments for children.

The goal of this conference is to enlist the help of all 300 invited participants in developing specific recommendations for a National Action Agenda for children's mental health. This conference represents an unparalleled opportunity to make a difference in the quality of life for America's children and adolescents. While the task ahead will not be easy, he emphasized the need to take advantage of "golden opportunities" which can often be "disguised as irresolvable problems."

STEVEN E. HYMAN, M.D., Director, National Institute of Mental Health

Dr. Hyman stressed how important Dr. Satcher's focus on mental health issues has been. Dr. Satcher has devoted much of his time to mental health, he said, and it has made an enormous difference. When the Surgeon General of the United States recognizes the centrality of mental health to all of health, there is an enormous change throughout the country. It is difficult to imagine anything more important than the mental health of our children.

There is a need to recognize that children are engaged in a process of development. What does it mean if a child is unable to attend in school, spends years sad, anxious and unable to learn?

Can children regain lost ground if untreated for two, five or eight years? We have spent so much time, appropriately so, on the physical health of children. In education, cognitive development has been emphasized. In contrast, social and emotional school readiness has been pushed under the rug, or perhaps lost in debate over what we really know, who is responsible for what, and what impact is from parents, peers, and the community. In the meantime, our understanding of the social and emotional factors that provide for school readiness and for healthy development has lagged. More research is needed, but at the same time, much is known. There is a terrifying gap between what we do know and how we act, between the services we could offer and those we offer, and between what families can afford and what families can access.

Stigma is an important factor. Parents are fearful about bringing the social and emotional difficulties of their children to the attention of medical professionals, perhaps afraid they may be blamed. Children are sometimes directly stigmatized by the cruelty of classmates. This is stigma squared. Dr. Hyman reminded conference participants that we are working against a politicized environment rather than in a purely medical environment. There are many people who would like very much to have a referendum on the use of psychotropic drugs in children, he said. Yet, the real issue is appropriate diagnosis and treatment of our children. Do we have access to those treatments and to that care? What are the qualifications of the people to whom we bring our children? Have they been educated in these areas? How thorough is the investigation into what might be going wrong in a child? Does the practitioner have the training, the time, the financial resources to interact with the child, to talk to the family, to engage the family, to talk to the school, the daycare centers, and really understand what is going on? Do we have, too often, because of problems of access and problems of finance, an emergency room or a crisis mentality? In this conference, we have the opportunity to focus on the core issues that are going to affect the health of children.

BERNARD S. ARONS, M.D., Director, Center for Mental Health Services

Dr. Arons described the Center for Mental Health Services, which was formed eight years ago and whose mission is to improve the delivery of mental health services. The center, through block grants and Knowledge, Development and Application (KDA) grants, has funded projects on a wide variety of issues, including homelessness and job performance. KDA grants were used to pioneer systems of care for children with serious emotional disorders—a concept that changed the paradigm for delivering services to American children and their families.

The essential role of families in the care of those with mental illness is critical. The Center hammers away at barriers to care, Dr. Arons said. But progress is slow. Access and cultural competence are important issues. The center is trying to construct a bridge between science and treatment and back again. Prevention is critical. There is a critical need to intervene sooner. Dr. Arons provided an analogy of a surfer, treading water out in the ocean waiting for the right wave to come along. That wave is here, particularly for children's mental health, he said.

Each of the participants in this conference has been carefully chosen because of contributions he or she has made to the mental health of children. Many American children and families are not getting the help they need. What should be done to improve the way children with mental illnesses are served? The conference organizers look forward to

the participants helping to move children's mental health to the next steps.

Panel 1: Identifying, Recognizing and Referring Children with Mental Health Needs

CHAIR: Mary Jane England, M.D., Washington Business Group on Health

This panel approached the prevalence of mental health need from a variety of perspectives, revealing the broad picture of unmet needs, health disparities, and policy implications. It examined the discrepancy between need and availability of mental health and substance abuse services, integrating the multiple systems involved (e.g., juvenile justice, child welfare, substance abuse, special healthcare, etc.). It also weighed the pros and cons of labeling children with disorders, comparing diagnosis versus functional impairments from a developmental perspective. The panel also answered critical questions on how mental health needs are identified or recognized in various systems and the barriers to recognition. For example, how well do these systems identify and refer children with recognized mental health needs? What linkages do or do not exist among these systems? The various speakers provided national data on identification, recognition, and referral within these systems and identified, where appropriate, federal or state policies that address recognition, linkage, and treatment services.

IDENTIFICATION OF MENTAL HEALTH NEEDS

David (Dan) R. Offord, M.D.,
McMaster University

Dr. Offord presented a framework for why the nation needs to address mental health needs in children and adolescents. The burden of suffering of children with mental disorders is significant. In the United States, between the ages of 1 and 19, the group of conditions that lowers quality of life and reduces life chances the most are emotional and behavioral problems and associated impairments. No other set of conditions is close in the magnitude of its deleterious effects on children and youth in this age group. Children with these disorders are at much increased risk for dropping out of school, and of not being fully functional members of society in adulthood. This burden of disease includes the prevalence of mental illness, morbidity, and cost. All sectors of society are involved. Prevalence estimates range from 17.6 to 22 % (Costello, et al., 1996) in one study, and 16 % in another (Roberts, et. al., 1998). Furthermore, child mental disorders persist into adulthood; 74% of 21 year olds with mental disorders had prior problems. The cost to society is high in both human and fiscal terms.

To ensure their businesses will flourish, the business community understands that they need to reduce the casualty class, that is, children with early-breaking emotional and behavioral problems and associated difficulties. There is a need to come up with programs to raise the life quality for large groups of children. Criteria for child psychiatric disorders need to include not merely emotional or behavioral abnormality but to consider functional impairment as well. The frequency of mental health problems is highest among the very poor, but most children with mental health problems are from the middle class. Important issues to consider are risk factors and protective factors, as well as comorbidity of disorders, which is very common.

Patterns of service use are not well understood. According to the Great Smokey Mountains Study, one in five children used specialty health services in the last three months, and early termination of treatment is a problem (Costello, et al., 1996). Reasons for underutilization are unclear. Possible reasons may include stigma, cost, and parental dissatisfaction with services. More research is needed to understand the reasons for under-utilization and to increase compliance. It is not clear that services for children's mental health disorders are underutilized. In fact, there are long waiting lists for these services. There are, however, two issues. First, specialized children's mental health services alone will never be sufficient, by themselves, to reduce the tremendous burden of suffering from child mental disorders. What are needed, in addition to effective clinical services, are effective universal and targeted programs. Hopefully, this strategy will reduce the size of the population needing clinical services. All three intervention strategies—universal, targeted and clinical—should operate in the context of a civic community. Since clinical services are relatively scarce and very expensive, they should be targeted to children who need them the most, and are most likely to benefit from them.

Suggestions for a national agenda include: (1) Ensuring a community focus in developing the national action agenda; (2) Using a population approach; (3) Creating common intake mechanisms; (4) Collecting data, not just at the national and state levels, but at community levels as well; (5) Utilizing evidence-based interventions and keeping frontline workers up to date; (6) Using graded interventions (e.g., trying parent training as an inexpensive start); and (7) Underlining the importance of the first five years to ensure that when children start school, the race is fair.

Senora D. Simpson, Dr. PH.,
Family Member

Dr. Simpson provided a parent's perspective on the state of children's mental health in the United States. Every program professes to value parents, but with a caveat: "Don't get too involved or provide too much input, for we are after all the experts." Multiple barriers to access and communication difficulties among the multiple systems exist; parental involvement, family satisfaction, preferences and quality of life are often disregarded. There are a plethora of programs, laws, regulations, federal and state mandates, but many have conflicting or rigid rules, gaps in services, and arbitrary eligibility requirements that exclude treatment for comorbid problems (e.g., substance abuse). Rigid, invalid, outdated and culturally incompetent assessment tools obstruct early identification and treatment. Stigma continues despite congressional efforts. Quality, evidence-based treatment is limited to a few narrowly-defined populations or is not available. The sense is that profitability drives treatment decisions, not model practice. "In reality, humane services are often not available if one's pedigree is not acceptable." Very often the most in need do not get the services. Real parental involvement, and attention to family satisfaction, family practice and quality of life is often left to chance

Dr. Simpson noted that in her experience of dealing with several generations of family members with mental health problems, it is no easier to get help in the 1990s than in the 1960s. "Besides, it costs more now to get a worse outcome." She noted limited change in practice with cost containment. Suggestions for change

include: (1) Implementing evidence-based practice in mental health; (2) Charging federal governmental agencies to review legislation and regulations which impact early identification, referral, comprehensive and coordinated treatment for children's mental health; the goal of this review is to resolve duplications, and ameliorate conflicts and gaps in treatment services; (3) Moving beyond basic research into applied research, in particular normative and evaluation research; (4) Engaging professional organizations and educators to develop standardized models of higher education to produce high quality care providers; and (5) Increasing accountability for outcomes that are relevant within a broader context.

PRIMARY CARE AND IDENTIFICATION OF MENTAL HEALTH NEEDS

Kelly J. Kelleher, M.D., M.P.H.,
University of Pittsburgh

Dr. Kelleher reviewed practice in primary care, discussed efforts to improve identification, and considered policy options to improve the recognition and referral of children in primary care with mental health needs. Each year, there are more than 150 million pediatric visits to primary care providers in the United States (NAMCS, 1998). Primary care practitioners prescribe the majority of psychotropic drugs, and they often counsel families about behavior and emotional problems and disorders. Still, some surveys suggest that families do not view this counseling from family doctors as mental health services, even though the physicians do. Most children with mental health problems see their primary care providers rather than mental health specialists. For many preschool children, such visits are their only contact with any major delivery system. Parents trust these primary care providers more than others. Yet, many barriers impede the delivery of effective mental healthcare. For example, the average visit is only between 11 and 15 minutes (NAMCS, 1988; CBS, 1997).

One major challenge is the disparity between what parents report versus what physicians report as psychiatric problems in children. In at least one large study, primary care physicians identified about 19% of all children they see with behavioral and emotional problems. Yet that overlapped by only 7% with what parents identified as problems. Girls and young children are less likely to be identified than boys. African American and Hispanic American children are identified and referred at the same rates as other children, but they are much less likely to actually receive specialty mental health services or psychotropic medications. This follow-through, or lack thereof, is very often linked to trust in the doctor, the history of that relationship, as well as demographics and insurance status.

Most referrals from primary care physicians for behavior problems are for child psychologists. Significant barriers to referral include lack of available specialists, insurance restrictions, and appointment delays. More than two thirds of primary care clinicians report appointment delays, with average time to appointment with a specialist being three to four months. Of those patients who were referred, 59% had zero visits to the specialist; only 13% averaged one or more visits a month in the follow-up period of six months. In short, an increasing number of problems (15-30%) are being identified by primary care providers, but rates of recognition (48-57%) are still low and connections to mental health specialists are difficult.

Dr. Kelleher suggested more efforts in the following areas: (1) Train primary care practitioners; this seems to have no impact on management practices except for those who

complete at least a two-year fellowship training. Nonetheless, the training of primary care physicians also needs to be expanded to include more mental health issues. (2) Screen for disorders in primary care; however, the effectiveness of screening depends on the availability of assistance for scoring screening protocols and the availability of treatment services. (3) Link specialty services through consultation-liaison services, co-location with mental health services, and use of behavioral specialists.

Public policy options include: (1) Payment coordination to ensure reimbursement for behavioral services by primary care providers, care coordination, parallel incentives for Managed Behavioral Health Organizations, Managed Care Organizations, and Primary Care Practitioners; (2) Data coordination through the Substance Abuse and Mental Health Administration (SAMHSA), Maternal and Child Health (MCH) Block grant requirements, Medicaid waiver requirements for sharing data, and state contract mandates, so that systems can track families and use reasonable case management across populations; (3) Accountability standards for screens, referrals, and treatment; and (4) Expansion of the Early and Periodic Screening, Diagnosis, and Treatment (EPSDT) program.

SCHOOLS AND IDENTIFICATION OF MENTAL HEALTH NEEDS

Steve Forness, Ed.D.,

University of California, Los Angeles

Dr. Forness pointed out issues specific to mental health needs within the school system. Children with mental health needs are usually identified by the schools only after their emotional or behavioral problems cannot be managed by their regular classroom teacher. A series of parent conferences, discipline referrals, or trial interventions in the regular classroom may precede formal referral to special education. Under the Federal Individuals with Disabilities Education Act (IDEA), such children should be formally evaluated and, if found eligible, either placed in a special classroom or provided special assistance in their regular classrooms. The five largest categories of special education include: learning disabilities (LD), speech and language handicaps (SL), mental retardation (MR), other health impaired (OHI) and emotional disturbance (ED). Learning disabilities and speech and language handicap count for the majority of the 11% of school age children in special education. Fewer than 1% of children are found eligible in the school category of emotional disturbance. Compared to children in the two largest categories of special education (LD and SL) who are mostly mainstreamed (over 80%), fewer than half the children under the ED category are mainstreamed.

A study done by Dr. Forness and a colleague in California showed that the schools are doing a very poor job of identifying children, or at identifying them soon enough. Among the thirteen year-old children from 12 special classrooms for children with emotional disturbance were diagnoses such as depression (approximately one third), attention deficit hyperactivity disorder (approximately one fourth), and post-traumatic stress disorder secondary to abuse. Before these children got into special education, parents reported recognizing a problem at a mean age of 3.5. Outside agency records (e.g., discipline referral, prescription medication) indicated problems at a mean age of 5 (i.e., kindergarten), and the first documented intervention involving some sort of pre-intervention was at age 6.5. The first eligibility for special education was at about 7.8 years (i.e., toward the end of second grade), and in more than 50% of the cases, these children were placed in the category of LD, not in the category of ED. These children finally got the right services at age 10.

In another long-term study of about 3,700 children done with his colleagues at the University of Alabama in Birmingham, assessments were conducted and mental health needs were identified using two diagnostic analogs of risk for emotional or behavioral disorders. Here again, the vast majority of these identified children did not receive special education services. Among those who did, a small minority were identified in the category of ED. Most were primarily categorized under the LD with a few in the SL category, even when controlling for those kids with comorbid diagnoses of learning, speech or language problems.

Dr. Forness pointed out that one of the major barriers to identification lies in the seriously flawed definition of ED. As a consequence, many children in need are deemed ineligible because of technicalities in the school definition of ED, and a significant number appear to be misidentified in other categories of special education reserved for children with primary learning or language disorders. This may be due to school professionals' or parents' attempts to avoid the stigma of mental health disorders or problems in appropriate detection or recognition of such disorders. In either case, under-identification or misidentification may also make it less likely that such children will be referred to other agencies for needed mental health services. Cost efficient systems for school mental health screening and methods for training regular and special education teachers in early detection of mental health disorders are available but seldom used effectively, if at all, in actual school practice.

Suggestions from Dr. Forness include: (1) Train school professionals, especially classroom teachers, to recognize early symptoms of emotional and behavioral disorders; (2) Modify the school definition of mental health disorders, which is more restrictive than definitions for other school categories; and (3) Develop a more proactive identification process for mental health disorders in school, in which children are screened for emotional or behavioral disorders early in the school years, just as they are screened for visual acuity or other health problems.

PRESCHOOL AND IDENTIFICATION OF MENTAL HEALTH NEEDS

Neal Halfon, M.D., M.P.H.,
University of California, Los Angeles

Dr. Halfon noted in the past several years that there has been an increasing policy focus on young children with two White House conferences as well as several foundation and government reports, which all highlight the importance of early childhood on brain development. An important finding of these reports is that plasticity decreases as people get older. He then used this fact to create a context for his further remarks.

Dr. Halfon suggested that the public policy context for understanding the development and identification of mental health needs in children must consider a couple of issues. First, from a public policy standpoint, he pointed out the contradiction in our current public investment in human capital (increasing social spending with age) with data portraying changes in brain plasticity, which demonstrates decreasing plasticity over the life course. What he suggested is that we are spending too little too late and missing an important opportunity to invest early. From the standpoint of prevention, early identification and treatment of mental health problems, we really need to talk about a new investment strategy in children's well-being.

The second contextual issue relates to the need to view things from a developmental perspective. Drawing on a life course health development

perspective, he suggested that experiences during sensitive periods of development have important long-term impact over the life course. Dr. Halfon introduced the notion of five developmental T's: trajectories, timing, transactions, transitions and turning points to highlight important implications for early identification and intervention. He suggested developmental trajectories for mental and behavioral function depend on the timing of experience and the character of the transactions between children and their caregivers. He also suggested that during transitions and turning points, such as the move from family care to childcare or childcare to preschool, children need extra support.

What do we know about young children? From a limited number of studies, mental health disorders in young children show similar prevalence rates to those found in older children. The catch is that you have to look more carefully to find them. Moreover, studies indicate there are high rates of stability of disorders especially for externalizing disorders that include disruptive behaviors and more aggressive kinds of behavioral problems. We also know there are sub-threshold behavioral problems that are identifiable and predictive. Increasingly, research has shown that a number of biological markers that can be identified early in a child's life have predictive power for the development of future problems. However, a majority of problems go unrecognized and most children do not receive treatment early in their life unless these problems are severe.

There are several types of risk factors for the development of mental health problems. There are a number of social factors that have been associated with the development of mental health problems, and poverty has been demonstrated to be an important risk factor in the younger years. National data indicate that 22% of children between the ages of 0 to 5 live in poverty, which represents a sizeable exposure to a potent risk factor. There are also biological factors (prematurity), family factors (resources, capacity, stresses and supports), and parenting issues (responsiveness and sensitivity of care givers, and mental health of caregiver) that pose risks.

In addition to highlighting the risk that many children face, evidence indicates that we are missing many opportunities for prevention and intervention. Few young children are recognized to have mental health and behavioral problems and most do not receive appropriate and timely treatment. Dr. Halfon suggested that we have a major gap between research and practice. Thus, interventions that have been shown to be effective are not widely utilized. We also have no national data on prevalence, trends and access, and quality of services that are specifically focused on young children. The only national health data source available is the National Health Interview Survey, and it is very difficult to get any reliable estimates for children under five years of age from this data source. Dr. Halfon also suggested that our deficiencies in collecting data on prevalence, impact, and provision of appropriate services were imminently correctable. A number of effective preventive mental health services for young children exist, such as home-based, center-based programs and community-wide programs; but these are not widely applied.

In terms of pediatric practices, a national study conducted by Dr. Halfon found that routine developmental and psychosocial assessments of young children and their families using standardized instruments are rarely used in pediatric practices, and when psychosocial screening is conducted by pediatric providers it is associated with available community resources. Pediatricians do not screen for maternal depression, or important risk factors for the development of childhood mental health problems, if there is no place to send those mothers for appropriate treatment. Another limitation of pediatric primary care relates to training pediatricians to conduct psychosocial screening and the importance of developing new tools to make such screening more effective and efficient.

Suggestions for public policy include (1) Create a context for child mental health policy and one that looks at how we invest in the lives of young children; (2) Include mental health prevention and the promotion of socio-emotional development in statewide early childhood initiatives; (3) Revolutionize pediatric care, including new assessment measures and protocols, new standards and guidelines, local-area developmental-resource networks that include services for entire families, appropriate reimbursement, quality measurement and accountability; (4) Institute more appropriate national data on families with young children either through the expansion of the National Health Interview Survey or the new Maternal Child Health Bureau's proposed survey; and (5) Conduct systematic monitoring of access and quality specifically around prevention services, treatment services, and community-wide services.

Suggestions for research include (1) Development of longitudinal population studies of developmental determinants of psychopathology; (2) Expansion of integrative clinical research on gene-environment interactions; (3) Intervention and practice research; and (4) Prevention research, at a community level, which takes advantage of community systems, coordinating efforts across the National Institute of Mental Health, the Maternal and Child Health Bureau and the Centers for Disease Control.

CHILD WELFARE AND IDENTIFICATION OF MENTAL HEALTH NEEDS

John Landsverk, Ph.D.,

Children's Hospital, San Diego

Dr. Landsverk reviewed the mental health needs specific to the foster care system. Research studies over the past two decades have firmly established that children in foster care represent a high-risk population for maladaptive outcomes, including socio-emotional, behavioral, and psychiatric problems warranting mental health treatments. Recent studies in California, Washington State and Pennsylvania suggest a high use of mental health services by children in foster care, largely due to linkage to Medicaid funding. But, it is important to note that foster care is not a mental health system.

The number of children in the welfare system can be best estimated from the number of children in foster care. 1995 estimates place that number at 482,000 to 710,000. This number should then be multiplied two or three times to account for children who are reported to child protective services and children receiving in-home services. Entrance into this system occurs when a child is maltreated; neglect is the most common reason (50-60%), followed by physical abuse (20-25%), sexual abuse (10-15%) and physiological/medical neglect (5-10%). The largest group is a young population, ages 0 to 5, poor, minority, in female head of household homes. This young group enters the system at roughly twice the rate of children ages 6 and older. Foster care children represent an extremely high-risk population. Half of the children (ages 0 to 17) in foster care have adaptive functioning scores in the problematic range; among children ages 0 to 6, 50-65% are in the problematic range in terms of developmental status; among 2 to 17 year olds, 50-60% have behavior problems; and among the 6 to 17 year olds, about 40% meet the criteria for any diagnosis with moderate impairment.

In terms of mental health service use, children in foster care use these services up to fifteen times more than other children in the Medicaid system. Foster children with behavioral problems are most likely to be seen. Data also show that children with a history of sexual abuse are three times more likely to receive mental health services, while children with a history of neglect are only half as likely to receive treatment. African-American and Hispanic children are least likely to receive services, and they need to display more pathology to be referred for mental health services. Developmental services are accessed significantly less than would be expected based on the high rate of developmental problems observed.

Despite the large mental health service utilization in the child welfare system, the use of evidence-based treatments is very low, and the dominant focus of treatment is on sexual abuse and somewhat on physical abuse. In spite of the clear evidence that the long-term effects of neglect are equally as damaging, there is almost no attention to this issue. Little is known about how effective services are for children involved in the child welfare system who remain with their biological parents. Promising evidence-based interventions include (1) Identification of developmental problems (Leslie, San Diego). (2) Foster Parent Management Training (Chamberlain, Oregon and San Diego). (3) Multi-systemic treatment for Physically Abusive Parents (Swenson, South Carolina). (4) Attachment intervention for foster parents (Dozier, Delaware). (5) Treatment Foster Care (Farmer, North Carolina). (6) Culture/Climate of Case Worker Teams (Glisson, Tennessee).

Suggestions for policy initiatives: (1) Expand use of the EPSDT Program to include comprehensive assessments; given the rates of problems, comprehensive assessment, rather than screening for problems, is the key issue. (2) Expand the use of the State Children's Health Insurance Program (SCHIP) funding streams to improve use of systematic assessment and evidence-based treatments.

JUVENILE JUSTICE AND IDENTIFICATION OF MENTAL HEALTH NEEDS

Linda A. Teplin, Ph.D.,
Northwestern University Medical School

Dr. Teplin discussed what can happen when the primary care, school, child welfare and the larger mental health systems fail. She suggested that changes in systems (e.g., Medicaid reductions, rise of managed care) have resulted in fewer children getting treatment for mental health problems. Consequently, many children are falling through the cracks and these kids are ending up in the juvenile justice system. Poor children, minority children, and children with comorbid disorders are disproportionately represented.

The literature suggests high rates of alcohol, drug, or mental (ADM) disorders in the juvenile justice population. Yet there are few empirical studies. There is even less information on ADM comorbidity among juvenile detainees, although related literature suggests rates may also be high. Dr. Teplin presented data from a study from Chicago that looked at the prevalence of mental disorders among children in a typical detention center. Among a sample of 1,829 children (650 girls), two thirds tested positive for drugs (although only 6% tested positive for drugs other than marijuana). Nearly three quarters of the females and over two thirds of the males had one or more psychiatric disorders. Nearly 20% of the sample had an affective disorder; rates were higher among females (27.5%). Comorbidity is common. For example, over two thirds of youth with an affective disorder also had substance abuse/dependence (alcohol, drug, or both). In addition, mortality is high. To date, 33 youth (1.8% of the sample) have died, all violently.

Based on these findings, the implications for policy and research are multiple. Correctional healthcare, particularly among juveniles, is a growing national public health problem. The magnitude of mental health service needs far exceeds current resources. Dr. Teplin and colleagues are doing follow-up interviews with the children in the study. "We are struck by the enormous proportion of our girls, only 10 to 17 at baseline, who are holding babies during the follow-up interview," she said. "Only if we provide services, innovative services geared towards the mental health needs of these kids, can we hope to break the cycle of disorder."

Recommendations to address mental health needs in the juvenile justice system include: (1) Reduce the number of children in the juvenile justice system by improving identification and services in other systems—primary care, schools, welfare and the larger mental health system. (2) Conduct research into understanding patterns of ADM comorbidity. It is central to providing effective interventions for high-risk youth both in the juvenile justice system and in their communities. (3) Take steps to improve mental health services for the children in the juvenile justice system. Adequate services would include screening and treatment, with attention paid to gender differences and comorbidity.

DISCUSSANTS

Donna Gore Olsen,

Indiana Parent Information Network

Ms. Olsen is a family member who represents several family advocacy groups, including the Family Voices and the Indiana Federation of Families. She emphasized the importance of quality, family-centered mental health services based on her own family's experience and those of other families. Ms. Olsen expressed concern that families' reports of problems, which they frequently recognize before anyone else, are often ignored or minimized. She urged the providers to talk to families and listen to their needs, be they related to chronic illness, blended families, single parenthood, or serious emotional needs. She called for family-centered programs that include the whole family in counseling services as part of the plan of care, pointing out that many of the programs tend to be only child-centered. Further, she pointed out the need for accessible programs, which sometimes means in families' homes, and programs that are coordinated across the multiple disciplines involved in a child's care. Often, confidentiality is used to prevent this necessary collaboration. Anecdotally, Ms. Olsen reported that the reason most families do not return for therapy appointments is because they have not received the practical information they need and want. Finally, she highlighted a neglected area, namely, transition programs to ease the stress of transition from pediatric to adult services for children with special healthcare needs.

Glorisa Canino, Ph.D.,

University of Puerto Rico

Dr. Canino highlighted a common theme in the presentations thus far: the lack of access to mental health services in different settings, particularly for minority children. The stigma of mental health problems is far greater for minority children. Some reasons for this disparity include lack of cultural competence of mental health providers and lack of outreach programs. The consequence is that many children end up incarcerated; many of these are minority children. Other important issues that need to be addressed include family burden, where family members are left caring for these problems on their own; the long-term consequences of untreated mental illness (i.e., adult psychopathology); and the impact of cost containment on service delivery.

Lucille Eber, Ed.D.,

The Illinois Emotional/Behavioral Disabilities Network, Riverside, Illinois

Dr. Eber noted the important role schools can play in identifying and intervening with mental health problems in children. However, schools are not experiencing much success, even with the small percentage of children identified. A primary issue is the lack of infrastructure in schools for providing proactive behavior supports around all students. Without universal conditions to improve behavior and academic learning for all children, effective interventions are less likely for the children with the greatest needs. A lack of comprehensive support systems and training for teachers and administrators have led to reactive, punitive, control/containment interventions that do not work to establish positive behaviors and improve learning. She cautioned, "Identification without quality intervention leads to chaos." She urged a rethinking of mental health models for schools. This includes moving beyond special education as the source of intervention and using mental health resources in a different manner than traditional clinical models. A comprehensive system of universal (school-wide), targeted (for at-risk students) and intensive and comprehensive interventions for those with complex problems is needed. This requires establishing more proactive host environments in the school. She commented on the need to change the current Emotional Disturbance definition, for increased training and staff development, and to change state certification requirements in order to impact the university training for teachers and administrators. New roles for social workers and school psychologists should be considered so that they can more effectively support students, teachers and families and create partnerships with the mental health, child welfare and juvenile justice systems.

Velma LaPoint, Ph.D.,
Howard University

Dr. LaPoint advocated a holistic, ecological approach to children's mental health in research, interventions, policy, and advocacy. She concurred with Dr. Senora Simpson about the need for professionals to meaningfully and proactively involve families in identifying children's mental health needs, developing, implementing, and evaluating interventions. Mental health educational materials that are linguistically and culturally relevant for families are also needed.

While Dr. Forness focused on children labeled as in need of special education, Dr. LaPoint focused on all students attending public schools. She stated that teachers need pre-service and continuing professional development on how to recognize indicators of children's mental health problems. Teachers need to be aware of new and continuing challenges to children's mental health (e.g., parental divorce or incarceration, advertising and marketing of targeted youth products, gun violence) and school systems need to support teachers by having high quality referral and school-based treatment systems, where appropriate, for children showing signs of mental health problems.

Equally important are issues of how school organization, classroom practices, and other related factors, including teachers' personalities and management skills, can influence children's behavior at school. There is also a need to go beyond the common signs of mental health problems and use indices such as chronic absenteeism that may be related to serious child mental health problems. A broad assessment of children's social competence, including their assets and support networks, is needed by educators so that programs can be developed, implemented, and evaluated to enhance their academic achievement and social competence. Adequate district, state, and/or federal funding are needed to provide schools with adequate counseling and related support services. There is a need to reduce the student-counselor ratio and to make better use of school counselors and psychologists. Student-counselor ratios across the country can range from 300 to 600 students to one counselor, with higher ratios in high schools and large urban school districts, generally serving low-income students of color. School counselors are often not engaged in counseling tasks, and may spend a great amount of time on bureaucratic tasks. School psychologists and educational psychologists may have tasks that primarily focus on student problem identification and placement as opposed to developing and evaluating new and creative educational programs that can both prevent and treat students showing signs of mental health problems. School systems need to revisit the roles of social workers and nurses who can also play a major role in developing mental health prevention and treatment programs.

Dr. LaPoint went further than Dr. Teplin to say that a number of children in the juvenile justice system are in fact, intentionally programmed or tracked to the juvenile justice system. Some research suggests that poor children and children of color are tracked into the juvenile justice system while their white, middle-class counterparts are diverted to health and mental health systems resulting in a two-tiered child mental health service delivery system. There is no need for this kind of service delivery system given the vast economic wealth of this country. The issue, for all stakeholders in our communities and society, including service providers and elected and appointed officials, is to have the political will to serve all children with equity in attitudes, practices, and resources.

Panel 2: Health Service Disparities: Access, Quality, and Diversity

CHAIR: Spero M. Manson, Ph.D., University of Colorado
ACCESS, BARRIERS, and QUALITY

Pathways into, through, and out of service systems are issues of critical importance when addressing access to care, adequacy or appropriateness of care, as well as quality. This panel addressed these issues, examining the impact of race, ethnicity, and cultural attitudes.

David T. Takeuchi, Ph.D.,
Indiana University

Dr. Takeuchi discussed the importance of race as a separate and independent factor in children's mental health status, as well as access to and quality of care. Over the past two decades, it has been common to advocate for a more universal approach to resolving the disparities found among racial groups. Despite one's position regarding whether race has or has not declined in significance in American society, an advocacy for policies that attempt to reduce socio-economic status (SES) differentials is seen as a more

effective public policy strategy to gain acceptance among all racial groups and, equally important, policy makers.

While this approach is popular and well meaning, it tends to ignore an evolving body of research that finds race to have a strong effect on mental health variables, independent of SES. For example, a recent study assessing health outcomes for 50 states found a strong association between racial composition and health. The greater the minority composition, the poorer the child health profiles. When race was included in analytical models, income and equality did not have a significant association with child health outcomes. Another significant variable linked to improved child health outcomes was the willingness of states to fund social welfare programs. These analyses suggest that simply focusing on income inequality will not resolve racism and its consequences. Racism is a continuous problem and creates a social environment characterized by alienation, frustration, powerlessness, stress and demoralization, all of which can have pernicious consequences on mental health. There are programs that are trying to make health systems more equitable through education and attempting to reduce stereotypes and prejudice by providing information about different racial groups. Research indicates, however, that individuals who have preexisting racist beliefs may actually have these beliefs reinforced through such educational programs.

In order to address ethnic and racial inequities in children's mental healthcare, racism must be viewed in a broader context, focusing on institutional racism and the racial hierarchy of society and its systems, including healthcare. It is unclear how to do this, but two examples to consider would be Native Americans' building casinos to address economic inequity; and Native

Hawaiians' current effort to achieve sovereignty. These are two natural situations in which it can be seen how health outcomes will be influenced.

Margarita Alegría, Ph.D.,

University of Puerto Rico

Dr. Alegría discussed challenges in advancing equity in mental healthcare for children of color. She presented three arguments for increased focus on racial and ethnic differences. First, race, ethnicity and culture of children play a major role in shaping the care provided to them by health institutions. Racial, ethnic and cultural differences influence the expression and identification of the need for services. Studies have shown ethnic and racial differences in youths' self-reports of problem behaviors, caregivers' value judgments of what is normative behavior and caregiver expectations of the child. Ethnic and racial bias in who gets identified, referred and treated within certain institutions has also been documented. For example, African American youth are more frequently referred for conduct problems or to corrections rather than psychiatric hospitals, even with lower or equal measures of aggressive behavior. Quality of care is also impacted. For example, ADHD is less often treated by medications in minority groups than in white populations. There is also increased probability of misdiagnoses among minority individuals, affecting subsequent care.

Second, there are challenges in identifying the mechanisms by which ethnicity, race, and culture account for disparities in behavioral and emotional problems and service delivery. Understanding these mechanisms has important implications for how to intervene correctly. Factors that mediate such challenges may be related to lack of early detection by providers and parents; untrained and culturally insensitive providers; and lack of parent and provider knowledge of efficacious treatments.

For example, Latino youths have the highest rate of suicide, yet they are less likely to be identified by their caregivers as having problems. Disparities in services may be due to different barriers such as insurance status and settings where mental healthcare is delivered. Minority children tend to receive mental health services through the juvenile justice and welfare systems more often than through schools or special settings.

Third, efforts to address racial and ethnic disparities in mental health and service delivery are constrained by profound socio-environmental, institutional, and market forces. For example, managed care, by targeting medical necessity, may be constrained in obtaining the complexity of funding streams that are necessary to service minority children in the schools, juvenile justice settings or welfare agencies. Expansion of Medicaid eligibility for near poor families may not prove sufficient to increase mental health service usage, if it is not tied to increased provider availability and provider payment incentives to treat minority populations within depressed inner-city communities. Thus, a critical analysis of how residential, institutional, and market policies may create disparities is needed, and more importantly, of how these policies are implemented in ways that result in disparities. There is a need to address these disparities by moving beyond the healthcare sector, examining neighborhoods where minority children live (areas of economic disadvantage, concentration of violence in certain areas), addressing the institutions with which minority children interact (i.e., the referral bias in the various systems); and addressing the role of managed care and the lack of culturally competent providers in the various systems.

Suggestions to address these disparities include: (1) Ensure that efforts focus not only on equalizing access to treatment, but also on equalizing outcomes of care; (2) Aggressively monitor institutional progress towards an equitable and compassionate system of mental healthcare for children of color; and (3) Move beyond policy interventions in the healthcare system to more socio-educational approaches, where government agencies are not agents of control but agents of support.

Kenneth B. Wells, M.D., M.P.H.,
UCLA/RAND

Dr. Wells presented new preliminary data from three national surveys on access to specialty mental healthcare. The findings demonstrated high levels of unmet need for specialty care for children and adolescents and substantial ethnic disparities in access to such care. Detailed findings will be presented in a forthcoming article. Dr. Wells also drew attention to key issues in formulating public policy to address unmet need for child services. One set of issues relates to children in the public sector, where differences within and across states in implementation of policies to cover uninsured children result in children with varying degrees of vulnerability to unmet need for mental healthcare. Policies that guarantee coverage for uninsured children across diverse populations and geographic areas are needed to address this problem. Another set of issues applies to the private sector, where there has been much debate about the feasibility of implementing parity for mental health and physical health services for both children and adults; yet prior studies suggest that children have more to gain from parity, as they tend to be high utilizers if they use services and more quickly reach plan limits on coverage (Sturm, 1997). Thus achieving parity of coverage in the private sector may be especially important for addressing unmet need for child mental health services. Yet, Dr. Wells indicated that the meaning of parity is changing under managed care, as the defined

benefit does not necessarily directly correspond to the level of care provided under management policies (Burnam and Escarce,1999). Finally, Dr. Wells provided an example of the promise of quality improvement for mental disorders for adults, Partners in Care; in that study, depressed primary care patients from clinics using quality improvement programs had better one-year clinical outcomes and retention in employment than similar patients in clinics without quality improvement programs (Wells, et. al., 2000). These kinds of studies should be developed for children and adolescents with major mental disorders, as we develop practice-based solutions across public and private sectors to address unmet need for diverse child and adolescent populations.

Suggestions for future research include:
(1) Develop access and mental health quality of care indicators for children and adolescents;
(2) Profile unmet need for under- and uninsured subgroups in particular areas, in light of disparity in coverage and implementation across federal and state programs; and (3) Monitor access and quality of care for children and adolescents nationally. Suggestions for policy changes include: (1) For the uninsured, replace existing programs or fill the diverse gaps in federal and state policies; (2) For the privately insured, start with parity of mental health coverage with medical conditions, and enforce tougher mandates for implementation. In addition, the management and quality under parity needs to be evaluated; and (3) For the publicly insured, implement quality improvement, and reduce delays and the financial barriers to mental healthcare.

REACHING OUT TO AND ENGAGING FAMILIES

This panel discussed the challenges affecting access to and coordination of mental healthcare for children and families, including the lack of availability of non-traditional services. One critical question addressed how to better engage families in evidence-based services and treatments.

Barbara J. Friesen, Ph.D.,
Portland State University

Dr. Friesen argued that effective mental health services require cultural competence, full family participation and appropriate services and supports. Family support and participation can provide benefits including reduced need for inpatient treatment, shorter length of inpatient stay, better service coordination, increased likelihood that a child will return home following out-of-home placement, and increased caregiver satisfaction. When families were involved in the child welfare system, they were more likely to follow through with treatment and the caseworkers were more likely to provide appropriate care.

There are several significant barriers to family participation and effective treatment for children's psychiatric disorders. First, stigma attached to mental disorders results in families feeling at fault for their child's mental illness. Low-income families are most likely to receive disrespect from healthcare providers. Second, family and service providers lack information. Third, gaps in services are a major problem. Even when a family is armed with information about exactly what they are looking for, very often they cannot find it. Other practical, tangible barriers include cost; many families have gone bankrupt trying to care for their children. The most damaging policy is one in which parents need to give up custody in order to

get services for their children. Distance can also be a barrier to care. Sometimes families must travel long distances to receive appropriate care for their child.

Suggestions for engaging families include: (1) Develop anti-stigma campaigns to educate the public and healthcare providers; (2) Train services providers in effective, family-centered treatment approaches; (3) Support family members and family organizations who can improve access to services through a variety of outreach and support roles; and (4) Evaluate these practices.

C. Vereé Jenkins
Family Involvement Coordinator, Family HOPE, West Palm Beach, Florida

Ms. Jenkins described her family's experience overcoming the ravages of the mental illness of her son, Joel. She called it the story of "J.O.E.L.: Joy Overcoming Everything Logical." She emphasized the importance of faith in dealing with a child's mental illness. Joel had a journey through mental illness, substance abuse, the juvenile justice system and early fatherhood. All along the way, no one ever asked the family their faith and what they believed in, said Ms. Jenkins. In a substance abuse treatment program, Joel had his bible taken from him, told it was a crutch preventing him from overcoming his substance abuse problems. But, Ms. Jenkins said, you need faith in God to make it through these systems; you put faith in the hands of the therapist managing your care and sometimes are let down. Finally, Joel went to the church where he found 'wrap-around faith' where they provided mentoring, counseling services 24 hours a day, seven days a week, helped him get a job and get rid of his guns and provided other assistance. Ms. Jenkins encouraged consideration of faith-based organizations, which can provide safe havens, camps, music, art, and all sorts of activities that can be very helpful to a family in need. Joel is now drug, alcohol and cigarette free. He is a law-abiding citizen, married, a good parent, employed and owns his home. A recent graduate of the McCollough Seminary, he is Assistant Youth Pastor of his church. As a family, Joel, Ms. Jenkins and her husband work together to share their faith and hope with others.

Lynn Pedraza, Ed.S.,
Family Member

Ms. Pedraza described how her family, which includes biological, foster and adoptive children, encountered many challenges trying to navigate the multiple systems often involved in the care and treatment of children with mental disorders. So much of the mental health world operates from a deficit perspective requiring families to prove their needs, rather than strengths, to get services. Workers have coerced parents and threatened to take children away when families try to fight for appropriate services. Suggestions to engage families include: (1) Put mental health at the forefront of health policy decisions and research efforts; (2) Research should focus on the human side of mental health, the connections to others, trust, pleasure, joy and respect. In other words, examine what caring looks like and what happens when this caring is incorporated into mental health services; and (3) Researchers need to become involved with families and their children long enough and deeply enough to really understand the multiple factors that affect children and their families. Researchers need to listen to families.

DISCUSSANTS

Brenda Souto,
National Alliance for the Mentally Ill

Ms. Souto described her experiences as a parent of a child with several disorders. She has been her son's case manager for 20 years and has had good experiences with psychiatrists and psychologists in Maryland, a parity-enforced state. Trying to find good services was another problem. She cited a report, *Families on the Brink*, that NAMI released a year ago, summarizing the stigmatization of families who often are blamed for no-fault brain disorders. She said the most unfortunate result of the lack of access to mental healthcare is when the family is forced to relinquish custody of their ill child to the state in order to get needed mental health services.

Carl Bell, M.D.,
Community Mental Health Council, Chicago

Dr. Bell described the insufficient infrastructure in the community health system. Back in 1980, President Jimmy Carter pushed for a plan to increase the infrastructure. But the plan never came into being because Carter lost the presidency. Dr. Bell encouraged conference participants to make sure they take action to ensure the agenda moves forward. He is particularly interested in African Americans. In order to fix the problems of African Americans within these various systems, African Americans must be involved in the conversations. The black community trusts the community centers but not the universities. Black people are concerned about who is testing their children and why. Partnerships between community-based organizations and the universities is one way to make technical expertise available to train community-based staff. Such efforts are underway at Dr. Bell's agency and the University of Illinois in Chicago, but they are costly. Few community agencies have the resources needed to train their staff in evidence-based interventions. Community-based organizations need to receive funding to assist them in training their staff and such support is necessary to help infuse evidence-based interventions into community-based services.

Michael M. Faenza, MSSW,
National Mental Health Association

Mr. Faenza noted this session's presentations demonstrate children's mental health as a social justice issue. The disparities in access and treatment highlight the social injustice issues that come into play in children's services. He highlighted challenges in diagnosing mental disorders in children, and a need for more research in diagnosis and treatment. Because so much negative public attention is focused on overprescription of psychotropic medications and overdiagnosis in young children, particular sensitivity around such issues is needed to prevent the damage that such publicity could do. The prevalence of mental disorders and substance abuse disorders in the juvenile justice system suggests a starting point for change in operative services systems for children.

Phillipa Hambrick,
Family Member

Ms. Hambrick described her experiences as a grandmother and mother, providing family care to four grandchildren in need of mental health services, for ADHD and major depression. She had difficulty getting services for these children, due to distance or because the children were put on a waiting list for services. The children eventually received services through the school system and through youth and family services. But such services must be expanded and made more comprehensive, she said. If she were to move, her children would lose the services because they would be in a different jurisdiction.

Panel 3: State of the Evidence on Treatments, Services, Systems of Care and Financing

CHAIR: Chris Koyanagi, Bazelon Center for Mental Health Law

PREVENTION, EARLY INTERVENTION and COMMUNITY-BASED SERVICES

This group examined the state of the evidence on effectiveness of services for youth with or at risk for persistent or multiple disorders, including respite care, wrap-around services, school-based treatments and others. The panelists looked at where the evidence is the strongest and where it is the weakest. They highlighted the gaps between what we know and what we are doing in a variety of areas.

Barbara J. Burns, Ph.D.,
Duke University

Dr. Burns highlighted reasons for hope regarding improved outcomes for children with severe, persistent, or multiple mental disorders. There is significant growth in the evidence base for interventions targeted towards the prevention and treatment of mental disorders; increased under-standing about changing clinical practice; tools for improving clinical practice; and policy to support implementation of some community-based interventions.

Although of recent origin, the published research of controlled studies can be examined to discriminate among interventions with strong, moderate, or weak evidence of effectiveness. Dr. Burns highlighted recent findings from the prevention and early intervention literature, focusing on David Olds' nurse home visitation program for high-risk (low income and unmarried) mothers and their infants. This study has shown multiple and long-term benefits for both the mother and the children at 15-year follow-up. These benefits include reductions in child abuse and neglect, and fewer arrests among the mothers; fewer arrests and convictions, less substance abuse, and fewer sexual partners among the adolescents. Cost savings from this study are estimated at $4 saved for every dollar invested. Savings are from child welfare costs, taxes on increased income, and reductions in criminal justice costs.

For youth who manifest severe emotional or behavioral disorders, the positive evidence for home- and community-based treatments (e.g., multisystemic therapy, intensive case management, treatment foster care) contrasts sharply with the traditional forms of institutional care, which can have deleterious consequences (e.g., inpatient psychiatric hospital, residential treatment, group home). The community-based interventions with an evidence base share the following six characteristics: 1) They function as service components in a system of care and adhere to system of care values (e.g., individualized, family-centered, strengths-based [not pathology-oriented] and culturally competent); 2) They are provided in the community, homes, schools, and neighborhoods, not in an office; 3) With the exception of multisystemic therapy and sometimes case management, the direct care providers are not formally clinically trained. They are parents, volunteers, and counselors, although training and supervision are provided by traditionally trained mental health professionals; 4) These interventions may operate under the auspices of any of the human service sectors (i.e., education, mental health, child welfare, or juvenile justice), not just

mental health; 5) Their external validity is greatly enhanced because they were developed and studied in the field with real-world child and family clients, in contrast to volunteers in university studies; and 6) They are much less expensive to provide than institutional care when the full continuum of care in the community is in place.

With evidence that outcomes for children and their families can be improved, the challenge is to translate these findings into clinical practice and policy. It will be important to apply knowledge on how best to change practitioner behavior, to encourage development and use of quality tools to guide clinical practice, to understand the impact of organizational cultures and context for sustaining therapeutic interventions with fidelity, and to augment or adapt interventions to facilitate organizational and/or community fit.

The next frontier for child mental health services also pertains to training practitioners in the evidence base and to reimbursement policies. Questions to consider include: Should programs that do not have an evidence base continue to be paid for? Consensus about which interventions have sufficient evidence for implementation may be required for policymakers to support reimbursement. There is also clear need to continue to study other interventions with promise but insufficient evidence of benefit. Creative thinking and a strong action plan will be necessary to shift treatment resources into the community, and to design models for relevant training to ensure high quality implementation. Thus, suggestions for next steps include: (1) Gain consensus about which evidence-based interventions to disseminate; (2) Increase understanding of methods for creating change in clinical practice; (3) Develop training and consultation for implementing change in practice; and (4) Pursue a logical sequence of research on prevention and treatment development, dissemination, and sustainability.

Tim Lewis, Ph.D.,
University of Missouri

Dr. Lewis described the current status of special education services for children and youth with emotional or behavioral disorders (EBD) who are currently served under the Individuals with Disabilities Education Act (IDEA). Bearing in mind the caveat that these children represent a wide range of disorders, age groups, and educational settings, best practices identified in the literature include: social skills instruction; academic achievement; family involvement, training and support; and functional behavioral assessment and positive individual plans. In addition, strategies to adapt and adopt these practices have been recommended, including continuous assessment and monitoring of progress, provision for practice of new skills, multicomponent treatment, and programming for transfer and maintenance. Yet, the evidence for the efficacy of such services is limited. Approximately 50% of students labeled EBD drop out of school; only 42% of those who remain graduate with a diploma. Post secondary outcomes are also poor, including multiple jobs, criminal behavior, and unemployment.

On a positive note, recent innovations have focused on building schoolwide systems of positive behavioral support to prevent emotional/ behavioral disorders, intervene early with those students who are at risk, and prevent extreme forms of behavioral challenges such as school violence. These promising practices focus on schools providing regular, predictable, positive learning and teaching environments, positive adult and peer models, and a place to achieve academic and social behavioral success. Common components of these practices include a systemic proactive approach across school settings and personnel with ongoing training and support; effective academic/pre-academic instruction; home-school collaborations; and school-agency collaborations. The move is away from punishment and exclusion, to more inclusive systems of positive behavioral interventions and support. Data from one school indicate that such positive support systems can dramatically decrease the amount of time students spend in school suspension, resulting in hundreds of additional available instructional hours and corollary academic growth.

In sum, schools can and should play a central role in the development of emotional and behavioral success. Suggestions to help schools in this role include: (1) Increase the school's capacity to develop children's emotional and behavioral success. Schools need assistance in the development and sustained use of systems of positive behavioral interventions and support; (2) Develop research strategies and agendas that incorporate multiple disciplines in addressing children's emotional and behavioral needs; and (3) Continue research on schoolwide systems of prevention/early intervention.

STATE OF THE EVIDENCE ON TREATMENTS FOR CHILDREN AND THE RESEARCH TO PRACTICE GAP
These three panelists synthesized the evidence on psychosocial, pharmacological, and combination treatments, paying close attention to the gap between research and practice in various settings and systems. Questions considered included: What is known about evidence-based treatments, why

such knowledge is not used, how knowledge can be made more relevant, and how practice can be changed.

John R. Weisz, Ph.D.,

University of California, Los Angeles

Dr. Weisz examined the question of whether psychotherapy works for children. He detailed data from meta-analytic studies indicating that usual care (i.e., treatment evolved from clinical practice and supervision, and not primarily from research) has very weak effects. Indeed, studies thus far suggest that usual care is on average, no more helpful than having no treatment. By contrast, evidence-based treatments (i.e., systematically tested treatments) demonstrate moderate treatment effects, comparable to those found in adult outcome research. These treatments are manualized, tend to be specific to the treated problems, and they are relatively durable, lasting up to 6 months beyond treatment termination.

A recent task force has identified specific treatments that have been systematically tested, including those for fears and phobias, anxiety disorders, depression, ADHD, and conduct problems/disorders. For example, well-established treatments for fears and phobias include reinforced practice and participant modeling. Cognitive behavioral treatments are probably efficacious for depression and anxiety. Behavioral interventions, including behavioral parent training and behavioral modification in the classroom are well-established for ADHD. For conduct problems, well-established treatments include behavioral parent training and video modeling for parents; a variety of probably efficacious treatments include anger control training, problem-solving skills training, multisystemic therapy (MST), delinquency prevention, and parent-child interaction treatment. MST has been used effectively to treat some of

society's most serious conduct problems among delinquent children in the juvenile justice system.

Despite the poor evidence for usual care in general clinical practice, and the more positive findings for evidence-based treatments, the latter treatments are generally not being used in regular clinical practice. These beneficial treatments are confined largely to universities and research clinics. There are multiple reasons why these more beneficial treatments are not making their way into clinical practice. First, there is no official stamp of approval for these treatments, nothing like the kind of certification tested medications receive from the FDA. As a consequence, the treatments may lack the widespread acceptance needed for adoption by providers. Second, public awareness of evidence-based treatments is limited. There is no agency or industry to publicize the scientific evidence for psychotherapy, nothing parallel to the pharmaceutical industry, which does such an effective job of publicizing medications. Third, dissemination is slowed by the fact that gaining expertise in most psychotherapies requires considerable hands-on training and supervision. Low reimbursement rates and the managed care system make it more difficult for clinicians to take time from their practices for additional training and supervision. Fourth, because most of the evidence-based treatments have been developed and tested primarily outside community practice settings, they may need to be adapted to facilitate adoption and everyday use in practice settings. Finally, there are few incentives for busy clinicians to make major changes in their current clinical practice patterns, and there are significant disincentives.

Suggestions toward bridging the gap between research and practice include: (1) A government or private organization should be created to identify and certify the psychosocial treatments that work, thus creating a process parallel to what the FDA does with respect to medications; (2) Mental health demonstration and service programs funded by government entities should all be required to have independent evaluation of outcomes to determine which programs actually do enhance mental health, and which programs need to be improved; and (3) Consumers of mental health services should be empowered with information; parents of children referred for treatment should be informed, prior to treatment, about the nature of any intervention proposed to them, and the evidence on whether that intervention works, thus permitting parents to make informed decisions regarding their children's care.

Peter S. Jensen, M.D.,

Columbia University and New York State Psychiatric Institute

Dr. Jensen reviewed the state of the evidence regarding medication and combined treatments for children with mental disorders. Substantial progress has been made in the last few years in conducting high-quality scientific studies of the role and benefits of medications for the treatment of childhood mental disorders. Consequently, a sizable scientific evidence base is becoming available to help providers and parents make informed choices about medication treatment options, whether such medicines are used alone or combined with psychotherapies. Advances in the medication treatments are especially heartening for several disorders, including ADHD, obsessive-compulsive disorder (OCD), and childhood anxiety disorders. In addition, major studies are currently underway to test the benefits of psychotherapeutic, medication, and combined treatments for ADHD, major depression, and OCD. Similar sizable trials and substantial efforts are also being conducted in the areas of youth bipolar disorder, autism, and other selected major mental disorders affecting youth.

Dr. Jensen pointed out that children often have complex problems. For example, the rule for ADHD in general is that these children very often have other coexisting disorders. It therefore makes sense that combined treatment is useful for these children to the extent that these combinations address children's multiple difficulties. Unfortunately, only one study, the NIMH Multimodal Treatment of Children with ADHD (the MTA study), has examined these issues. This study demonstrated that medication alone proved to be more effective than behavior therapy alone for ADHD symptom relief. However, combined treatment, though not more effective than well-managed medication for most children, provided better clinical outcomes than medication alone for children with complex co-occurring problems. Another important finding from this study indicated that the medication management used in the study far exceeded routine community care that included medication treatment. This greater effectiveness under optimal conditions appeared to be clearly related to the frequency of office visits, their duration, dose frequency, and school contact. Thus, in the MTA medication management approach, visits were 30 minutes, once a month, dosage was higher and more frequent, and teachers' input was solicited to guide medication adjustments. In contrast, in routine community care, visits averaged only 18 minutes, twice a year. Thus, despite progress in the scientific evidence, substantial gaps appear to exist between the manner in which medications are used in ideal research-based settings (and the resulting well-established benefits), and the manner or quality of their use in "real world" settings. Given that parents prefer a combination of behavior therapy and medication, research into effective ways to use psychosocial therapies with medication in "real world" settings is needed. Although substantial knowledge is now available on the short-term safety and benefits of many of the psychoactive medications, little information is available on longer-term safety and efficacy of most agents. Uncontrolled studies suggest that longer-term use is not harmful per se, but it is not clear that longer-term use is appropriate or necessary for all children.

To bridge the gap between research and real world practice, accurate information on evidence-based treatments, training initiatives for mental health and other professionals, and policy initiatives are needed. There is a need to understand barriers and "promoters" to the delivery of effective services. Whether or not efficacious treatments are used has to do with child and family factors, provider/organizational factors, and systemic and societal factors. Thus, if families are concerned about stigma or if they are unable to accept a certain type of treatment, services will not be "effective," if only because they are not used. Similarly, if providers do not have the training, the time, or are not reimbursed, efficacious treatments will not work optimally in the real world.

Thomas P. Laughren, M.D.,
Food & Drug Administration

Dr. Laughren discussed FDA's role in pediatric psychopharmacology, namely to assess development programs proposed to study the safety and the effectiveness of psychotropic treatments for psychiatric disorders in pediatric populations and to review New Drug Applications (NDAs) submitted to support drug claims for such disorders. Since FDA does not regulate the practice of medicine, it does not generally address off-label use, i.e., the use of approved medications for uses that do not have approved claims. This is a particular problem for children since most medications used in this population are off-label. There are relatively few psychotropic drugs approved specifically for the treatment of pediatric psychiatric disorders. These include drugs for

obsessive-compulsive disorder (Clomipramine, Fluvoxamine, Sertraline), ADHD (Methylphenidate, Amphetamines, Pemoline), Tourette's Disorder (Haloperidol, Pimozide), Mania (Lithium), enuresis (Imipramine), psychoneurosis (Doxepin), and various behavior problems (Haloperidol, Chlorpromazine). This small number of approved indications in pediatric psychopharmacology is problematic for clinicians because they do not have an evidence base to guide their treatment decisions for the majority of psychiatric disturbances and symptoms that confront them in pediatric patients.

FDA has long recognized this problem in pediatric pharmacotherapeutics, and has launched several programs over the past 20 years to attempt to stimulate interest in pediatric studies. Two recent initiatives, the 1997 FDA Modernization Act (FDAMA) and the 1998 Pediatric Rule, have been particularly important in stimulating greater interest in developing drug treatments for the pediatric population. The Pediatric Rule gives the FDA authority to require certain studies be done in children both for a new drug and for an already approved drug that a company plans to develop for a new indication in adults. FDAMA is a voluntary program that gives a financial incentive (additional 6 months of patent exclusivity) for companies to study both new and marketed drugs in children. Under FDAMA, nine written requests have been issued for three psychiatric disorders in pediatric patients, i.e., major depressive disorder, obsessive-compulsive disorder, and generalized anxiety disorder. Under the Pediatric Rule, studies have been requested for post-traumatic stress disorder, social anxiety disorder, mania, and premenstrual dysphoric disorder. Other conditions under consideration for issuing written requests and requiring studies under the Pediatric Rule include schizophrenia, panic disorder, conduct disorder and ADHD (under age 6).

A question that always comes up when the FDA invokes the Pediatric Rule or issues written requests under FDAMA relates to the appropriate age cut-off for the various psychiatric indications of interest in pediatric psychopharmacology. Recent data regarding psychotropic drug use in the preschool population (Zito, et al, 2000) have amplified the question of what specific diagnostic entities or possibly non-specific psychiatric symptoms in this age group might benefit from more systematic study. For example, although methylphenidate is approved only down to age 6, there is substantial use under that age. So one set of questions relates to whether or not diagnoses such as ADHD, major depressive disorder and others, that are well accepted in older children are meaningful diagnoses in these younger children. An alternative view is that much of the prescribing of psychotropics in preschool patients, especially for conditions other than ADHD, represents treatment of non-specific symptoms such as aggression or self-injurious behavior. If so, are these non-specific symptoms a reasonable target for a development program? The safety of psychotropic drugs is, of course, also a concern in children who are growing and developing, and hence perceived to be more vulnerable to drug effects. Current assessment methods are not well developed and preclinical models to assess possibly subtle developmental effects are inadequate. Moreover, the ascertainment of adverse events is a particular challenge, especially in preschoolers. Optimal approaches for studying the safety of psychotropics in children are needed.

In order for FDA to move forward with implementing the Pediatric Rule and FDAMA for pediatric patients with psychiatric disorders, especially in the preschool population, it is critical for the field to make progress in establishing the validity of diagnoses and the validity of studying nonspecific symptoms in this population; in

developing better assessment instruments, both for efficacy and safety; and in generally advancing the science of psychopharmacological research in pediatric patients.

Evelyn P. Green,
Family Member

Ms. Green provided a family perspective on the availability and use of evidence-based treatments for childhood mental disorders. She described obstacles in acquiring information about children's mental disorders. Despite the large body of knowledge regarding what treatments are effective for children, this knowledge is not readily available or accessible, she said. Parents rely on their primary care doctors for diagnosis and for treatment options. Yet, all too often, professionals do not have sufficient knowledge and make incorrect diagnoses, hence diminishing chances of access to evidence-based treatments. Parents frequently must do research on their own to find this information because the schools, pediatricians and other professionals whom they rely on are not knowledgeable. It is thus imperative that frontline professionals have accurate information about how to evaluate and diagnose children's mental health problems to increase children's access to evidence-based treatments.

Even when parents and professionals are aware of the evidence-based treatments, they face several hurdles in accessing them. These include the stigma associated with "labeling" a child with a mental disorder; professionals who are not knowledgeable about evidence-based treatments; and reluctance by the educational system to provide the support needed to implement such treatments, especially regarding educational accommodations and medication use. Parents blame themselves and fear criticism for "drugging their child." Parental struggles to make the best choices for their children are exacerbated by inaccurate and sensational media reports or when so-called experts go on television to claim that mental illnesses in children do not exist. Scientific evidence is available, but is overwhelmed by the stigma associated with mental illness. Stigma can be lessened with open dialogue so parents can access treatment without fear or shame.

Suggestions to overcome such barriers to evidence-based treatments include: (1) Collaborative efforts by federal agencies, researchers, providers, educators and advocacy groups to educate the public about science-based information regarding mental disorders in children; (2) Providing health professionals and educators with science-based information and holding them accountable for proper use of that information; and (3) Developing efforts to help parents become better educated about mental illness and to advocate for evidence-based treatments.

SYSTEMS OF CARE: FINANCING AND ORGANIZING SERVICE SYSTEMS

This group examined the structure of reimbursement systems and their impact on access to and use of mental health services from a variety of perspectives, including that of the consumer and successful public-private partnerships. They also detailed some of the key elements in implementing effective services in the community.

Sherry Glied, Ph.D.,
Columbia University

Dr. Glied described the complex system of mental health financing in the United States. Essentially, funds flow in two distinct ways: insurance-based funds, which are attached to individual children, and public program funds, which finance distinct services such as community mental health centers, schools, welfare, and justice agencies.

This dual system of financing raises several concerns because different funding streams are financing similar services in different settings. First, services may be duplicated, which generates a risk of cost shifting from one area to another as spending is reduced. A second concern relates to coordination of treatment, which is especially problematic for children with serious emotional disorders (SED) who use multiple systems. Data from an SED study in Westchester County, New York indicated that 92% of children served by a public service system used services from two or more systems, and 19% used services from four or more systems. On the other hand, this financing structure creates redundancy, which provides greater opportunities to catch and treat children, especially those who are uninsured. Such redundancy is very important if you consider that about half of the children with mental health problems are never treated.

Dr. Glied focused on insurance for several reasons. First, the insurance model is expanding. Many states are allocating public dollars into insurance type programs and capitating their public mental health programs. Second, opportunities for insurance are expanding through programs such as the State Child Health Insurance Program (SCHIP). Of the uninsured children eligible for SCHIP, it is estimated that about 15% have some mental health problem. Third, insurance and financing is important because moving money is a lot easier than changing practitioner behavior. The extent that financing can alter practices has important policy implications.

Child mental health is not expensive. Children constitute about 28% of the population, but account for about 14% of health expenditures, and only about 7% of mental health expenditures. In 1996, children with mental health problems spent an average of $984 on mental health treatment in the healthcare system, which averages out to $45 per child. Most of this money is spent on inpatient services (39%), followed by physician services (24%), drugs (22%), non-physician, emergency room, and hospital outpatient services (10%, 3% and 2% respectively).

This picture raises concerns in several areas. First, as the role of insurance expands, managed care coverage is more common than traditional indemnity coverage, which reimbursed physicians on a fee-for-service basis. Managed care often includes capitated payment, especially of primary care practitioners. Since about two thirds of visits with mental health problems are to primary care practitioners, the increase in capitation raises concerns about risk selection at the provider level. On the other hand, this concern may not be very important, since changes in funding of primary care practitioners do not appear to affect diagnosis very much. For example, funding streams directed specifically at the recognition of psychiatric disorders among children (e.g., EPSDT through Medicaid) have not increased rates of recognition of mental health problems in primary care.

A second area of concern is specialized behavioral health carve-outs, as they now cover mental healthcare for almost 80% of insured children with psychiatric disorders, with major cost savings associated (30-40%). The concern here relates to utilization of services, quality of services, cost shifting to other sectors (especially public programs such as welfare and juvenile justice), and coordination of services under a carve-out model. Another important concern with carve-outs is in the area of coordination between mental and physical healthcare, particularly when mental health diagnosis is occurring in primary care. On the positive side, evidence to date indicates that a carve-out model may operate like a system of care. Overall, while the effect of carve-outs has not yet been fully assessed, they are likely to have both advantages and disadvantages.

A third area of concern is out-of-pocket costs, with higher co-payments and deductibles associated with mental healthcare making access more difficult. Parity legislation may eliminate this concern. As well, managed care may serve as a substitute for high co-payments and deductibles that traditionally were used to limit mental health spending.

So what are the significant future risks or concerns that remain as insurance type organizations and reimbursement mechanisms have proliferated? One concern is with utilization review. Most plans today incorporate utilization review, which has been shown to negatively affect re-admittance and quality of care, particularly for mental health services. The insurance model itself is also associated with risks. Insurance works on an average, but there is a highly skewed distribution of healthcare costs among children. This raises concern about selection, high disenrollment rates for children with mental health problems, and the adequacy of care for the costliest children. Given data that indicates that the top 15% of children with a mental health diagnosis account for 60% of all mental health cost, rationing may happen at the expense of the sickest children.

In light of these concerns, suggestions include: (1) Exploring the potential consequences of carve-out plans for children's mental health and (2) Addressing the effect of the shift from a program model to an insurance model on uninsured children.

Robert M. Friedman, Ph.D.,

University of South Florida

Dr. Friedman provided a theoretical framework for "systems of care", defined as a comprehensive spectrum of mental health and other necessary services that are organized into a coordinated network to meet the multiple and changing needs of children and adolescents with severe emotional disturbances and their families. Systems of care are viewed as evolving entities, adapting to changing conditions and contexts. Research on the effectiveness of systems of care, as evaluated in the *Surgeon General's Report on Mental Health*, indicates important system improvements, such as reducing use of residential placements and achieving improvements in functional behavior. There are also indications that parents are more satisfied in systems of care than in traditional service delivery systems. The effect of systems of care on cost is unclear. Furthermore, services delivered within a system of care have not been demonstrated to result in better clinical outcomes than those delivered in a usual services system. More attention needs to be paid to the relationship between changes at the system level and changes at the practice level. Currently, a national evaluation of the Comprehensive Community Mental Health Services Program for Children and their Families is being conducted.

Theories of change are underlying assumptions that guide service delivery and evaluations, and are believed to be critical to achieving desired goals. A theory of change for a system of care should describe the manner in which the system and practice levels are connected. Determining the extent to which that theory is implemented with fidelity is an important but often neglected part of evaluations. What is often missing in systems of care is the translation of experiences of service recipients back to the service system, so that these experiences affect services, and hence the system and policy. Too often, research fails to build from the experience of those who receive services. Because systems of care are a complex and evolving phenomenon, intensive study using a

variety of research and evaluation methods is needed. In-depth, qualitative studies that examine the individual experiences of children and families, perspectives of multiple stakeholders, and theories of change are important as part of the evaluation.

What about the applicability of evidence-based treatments for systems of care? A recent review of treatment effectiveness suggests that the effectiveness of services, no matter what they are, may hinge less on the particular type of service than on how, when and why families or caregivers are engaged in the delivery of care. Family engagement is a key component in treatment participation and care, and the effective implementation of that care. Research indicates that effective treatments emphasize flexibility, comprehensiveness, capacity for individualization, and the importance of the clinician/patient relationship. Yet the very characteristics that are likely to make services effective make them more difficult to describe and evaluate. One issue involved in assessing the applicability of evidence-based treatments to systems of care is the degree to which the treatments have been tested on populations comparable to the diverse population served in systems of care. There are opportunities to develop and apply evidence-based treatments in systems of care. In particular, those treatments that prescribe principles and general processes but allow flexibility for adaptation to strengths and needs of individual children and families and those that involve families and practitioners in the development of the interventions, have produced encouraging results. These include intensive case management, wraparound services, and multisystemic therapy. Beyond these, few evidence-based treatments have been developed and tested with diverse populations in natural settings.

The children's mental health field is largely divided, not just between the practitioner community and the research community, but also among the practitioner community, the evidence-based intervention community and the systems of care community. Each has much to offer, but there is a gulf between them that needs to be reduced. An additional challenge is how to support the early stages of development of interventions in real world settings, and the subsequent testing of those interventions in the real world.

Angelique Harris,

19 year-old youth

Ms. Harris shared her personal experience with mental illness and the mental health system. She has been receiving mental health services since age 15. She has used various services in the mental health system, including inpatient hospitalization. She described terrible conditions during her inpatient hospitalizations, both short- and long-term. She questioned if anyone would send their child into such a system if they could picture what goes on behind those doors. In her experience, staff were irresponsible and adolescents were treated as "guinea pigs," and were placed on every kind of neuroleptic medication. She was told that she was inferior because of her mental illness, and would never be able to succeed independently. When she left her last inpatient hospital, she proved them wrong. With her support system, which includes her grandmother, she has been taking medication responsibly. She lamented the lack of good mental health services, which she believes exist, but are in short supply. She urged that children with mental illnesses be treated not as fragile beings, but as individuals with a handicap, who have willpower, and can survive and function with support.

DISCUSSANTS

Trina Osher, M.A.,

Federation of Families for Children's Mental Health

Ms. Osher described the dramatic shifts in the children's mental healthcare system over the past fifteen years. These shifts have occurred in terms of (i) where children and youth receive treatment, services and supports: from hospitals and long-term residential care to the community; (ii) what constitutes such services: for example mentoring programs, anger management, family supports; and (iii) who provides them: for example, teachers, foster home child care staff, paraprofessionals, probation officers, and even community volunteers. As a result of these shifts, realizing good outcomes for children and youth with mental health problems and their families requires providing mental health services and supports in a comprehensive, culturally competent, coordinated, community-based, family-driven system of care.

Despite these shifts, a corresponding shift in research has been slow to occur. There is an urgent need to more fully understand the complexities of how systems of care function, how they impact the growth and development of children, youth and families, and how they affect long term outcomes in terms of the quality of life. Traditional research designs and methodologies are not sufficient for addressing critical questions about what works and what helps to bring about positive change for children, youth and their families who live in complex communities, coping with many different and intersecting social, political, economic, and cultural forces, and who receive a wide array of treatments, services and supports from a wide variety of sources. Ms. Osher challenged researchers, families and youth, practitioners, and policymakers to create more effective ways of studying the delivery of mental health services to children, youth, and families in real life settings. She called for a community-based research agenda, where the daily challenges faced by practitioners and families form the foundation for setting research priorities and funding distribution. She believes that connecting researchers, families and youth, and practitioners will lead directly to real change in practice because research results would be more relevant and would not require translation to be understandable in settings where mental heath treatments, supports and services are delivered.

Jane Knitzer, Ed.D,
Columbia University

Twenty years ago, Dr. Knitzer wrote a book called *Unclaimed Children* about children and adolescents in need of mental health services. The presentations she heard today were both wonderful and sobering. She was delighted about how much we have learned since then about treatments and about the strength of family and consumer voices. Yet, she expressed concern that we are starting too late. She focused her comments on building a knowledge-based system to promote emotional wellness and resilience in infants, toddlers and preschoolers facing a range of challenges. Some young children have serious emotional and behavioral disorders. Too often, they receive no help or inappropriate help, despite epidemiological evidence that suggests similar prevalence rates for serious disorders in young children as in older children. Another large group of young children are at risk of developing serious emotional disorders (SED). They are in families affected by maternal depression, substance abuse, domestic violence, and other risk factors. Research tells us that the cumulative impact of these risks for young children can be severe. This means that to help these children, we have to help their parents either with intensive interventions

(combining parent treatment, parent-child relationship therapy and child-focused interventions) or, with prevention-oriented strategies.

Systems to promote emotional wellness in young children also need to use non-familial caregivers systematically as agents of change. Young children are spending increasing time in early childhood daycare settings, and yet, mental health supports in these environments are very hard to create and sustain. Designing systems to support the emotional development of infants, toddlers and preschoolers requires a conceptual framework that is different from that for older children. Such systems must be developmentally appropriate, family-centered and prevention-oriented. This means addressing three critical issues: (1) Funding issues: Funding mechanisms must support direct services to young children as well as relationship-based therapies and consultation to non-parental caregivers by mental health providers in a range of settings. (2) System disconnect issues: Two sets of system disconnects are critical. First, adult and child systems are difficult to connect, except through demonstration projects such as Starting Early Starting Smart. Second, systems that deal with children's mental health often lack expertise in child development and early childhood and family clinical issues. (3) Diagnostic issues: Diagnostic systems in place for older children do not work for young children, but Medicaid and other funding streams have not been flexible in trying out alternatives such as the Diagnostic Classification for Zero to Three. Similarly, access to mental health services too often hinges on a child having the SED label. This is inconsistent with the emerging science of risk and resilience and makes it difficult to develop meaningful prevention.

The time is ripe for a major national initiative on behalf of infant and early childhood mental health. Such an initiative should include: (1) incentives for collaborative planning and systems development among early childhood, mental health and other systems such as substance abuse; (2) funds to support direct and preventive services; (3) incentives for professional training in skills and competencies necessary for infant and early childhood mental health; and (4) research that capitalizes on emerging field-based strategies, such as the growing number of consultation models, to build the knowledge base about effective practice.

Early brain research tells us that the roots of emotional regulation and development, so crucial for life and school success, lie in the earliest relationships. Experience and some research tell us that too many young children are headed for trouble. We must end this disconnect between research and practice. Building the capacity for infant and early childhood mental health will not be a panacea. But, absent systematic efforts to promote prevention, early intervention and relationship-based treatment for this age group we will simply create the SED, juvenile justice and special education population of the future.

Mark Greenberg, Ph.D.,

Pennsylvania State University

Dr. Greenberg presented evidence to highlight the need for prevention. For example, a study he conducted indicated that 48% of children with behavior problems in kindergarten were already in special education by fourth grade. He urged conference participants to consider well-established, empirically-validated programs that have demonstrated symptom reduction in the areas of conduct problems, depression, and event related trauma (e.g., divorce, bereavement, school transitions). He referred to a report prepared for

CMHS on this topic (Greenberg, et. al., 1999). These effective programs have three important components. They (1) build cognitive and behavioral skills that are protective, (2) help families and children gain better emotional awareness and regulation, and (3) improve the relationships of children with their parents and peers. Dr. Greenberg highlighted opportunities to utilize effective models of prevention in integrated systems of mental healthcare. He emphasized the need for a system of care that integrates prevention services, which are relatively low cost, along with other services (early intervention and high-end, high cost services) into one seamless system. Steps suggested to integrate mental health into systems of childcare, education, and other key systems, include: (1) Effective training for teachers and child care workers in social and emotional development; (2) Effective training for mental health professionals in evidence-based prevention practices; (3) Information for consumers on effective preventive models; and (4) Removing the disincentives in insurance systems for prevention activities so that healthcare professionals, especially primary care providers and others in the community will have incentives to provide early mental health preventive services.

Michael L. Dennis, Ph.D.,

Chestnut Health Systems, Bloomington, IL

Dr. Dennis described his experience both as a behavioral health researcher and a parent of children with comorbid mental disorders and medical conditions. He echoed previous presenters' difficulties in accessing mental health services from the system despite his professional status. Based on personal experience with both the private insurance and Medicaid systems, he personally testified that these systems have a major impact on where, what and how much care his children received. Clinicians who worked together in a biopsychosocial team were not the norm, and his family had to travel three hours to receive such service.

Dr. Dennis highlighted key points made by the panelists. Dr. Burns reminded us that "evidence-based" does not mean that it has to come from a medical or behavioral laboratory. In fact, several of the most effective interventions (e.g., MST) have evolved out of practice and been rigorously evaluated. Moreover, responses to many of the issues raised by Dr. Friedman about systems of care (e.g., placement, continuing care) almost have to come out of practice instead of the laboratory. While most research has been done in temporary or academic clinics, most treatment is done in such systems of care.

Dr. Weisz demonstrated the lack of effectiveness data on current practice, the promise of several evidence-based protocols, and reminded us of the limited number of studies that have been done. Dr. Weisz focused on the importance of manualized therapy. Dr. Dennis agreed, but thinks that the real common ingredient of these programs is actually the emphasis on quality assurance. Training with or without a manual has little impact. It is only real implementation and consistent delivery that lead to the kinds of effects found in these studies. His recent Cannabis Youth Treatment study demonstrated that serious quality assurance can be done with the cost and levels of resources associated with existing programs.

Dr. Jensen demonstrated that it is more than just having an effective medication. The medical protocol he found so effective was a behavioral medicine protocol that involved a lot more clinical time, follow-up and follow-through. The addition of behavioral components did not impact the ADHD symptom relief, but was key when there were multiple other problems and was preferred by

parents. This and the horror stories described by Ms. Harris, also remind us that quality assurance is important in both medical and behavioral protocols.

While much of the conference has focused on primary care and schools, Dr. Dennis reminded us that mental health problems exist in other specialties such as welfare, criminal justice, and substance abuse treatment agencies. For example, while the literature indicates that over 80% of adolescent substance abusers have multiple mental health problems, there is only token screening in most agencies. The number of adolescents presenting for adolescent marijuana treatment has doubled from 1992 to1998. One out of five adolescents are smoking the equivalent of 20 or more joints a day. Severity of marijuana use is directly correlated with increased attentional and violence problems and asthma. Further, over 20% of these adolescents drink to the point of blacking out and/or use hallucinogens like LSD, both of which exacerbate mental health problems. The official record typically documents about 10% of adolescent substance abusers as having mental health problems; about 8% have ever seen a mental health specialist and few services are available even for those. This is unacceptable. We need systematic screening of these special populations, integrated services and evaluations of how well protocols work with individuals with multiple problems, not just a single problem.

Dr. Dennis expressed hope that as we move forward with this agenda, we will broaden our approach to better address this comorbidity, improve the identification of mental illness among substance abusers and vice versa, improve access to care, and evaluate the effectiveness of treatments for individuals with both sets of problems—who represent the bulk of our system of care.

Appendix A

References

Burnam, M.A. and Escarce, J.J. (1999). Equity in managed care for mental disorders. Health Affair, 18(5): 22-31.

CBS 1997: Unpublished data from NIMH Grant MH50629: Management of Psychosocial Problems in Primary Care. Principal Investigator: Kelleher, K.

Costello, E.J.; Angold, A.; Burns, B.J.; Erkanli, A.; Stangl, D.K; and Tweed, D.L. (1996). The Great Smokey Mountains Study of youth: Functional impairment and serious emotional disturbance. Archives of General Psychiatry, 53(12): 1137-1143.

Greenberg, M.T.; Domitrovich, C.; and Bumbarger, B. (1999). Preventing mental disorder in school-aged children: A review of the effectiveness of prevention programs. Report submitted to The Center for Mental Health Services (SAMHSA), Prevention Research Center, Pennsylvania State University.

NAMCS 1998: Woodwell, D.A. National Ambulatory Medical Care Survey: 1998 Summary. Advance data from vital and health statistics, No. 315. Hyattsville, MD: National Center for Health Statistics 2000.

Roberts, R.E.; Attkisson, C.C.; and Rosenblatt, A. (1998). Prevalence of psychopathology among children and adolescents. American Journal of Psychiatry, 155(6): 715-25.

Sturm, R. (1997). How expensive is unlimited mental health care coverage under managed care? Journal of the American Medical Association, 278(18): 1533-7.

Wells, K.B.; Sherbourne, C.; Schoenbaum, M.; Duan, N.; Meredith, L.; Unutzer, J.; Miranda J.; Carney, M.F.; and Rubenstein, L.V. (2000). Impact of disseminating quality improvement programs for depression in managed primary care: a randomized controlled trial. Journal of the American Medical Association, 283(2): 212-20.

Zito, J.M.; Safer, D.J.; dosReis, S.; Gardner, J.F.; Boles, M.; and Lynch, F. (2000). Trends in the prescribing of psychotropic medications to preschoolers. Journal of the American Medical Association, 283(8): 1025-30.

Appendix B

Policy Brief

Title II of the Social Security Act, **SSI (Supplemental Security Income) Disability Benefits**, includes benefits for children. Supplemental Security Income is based on the following definitions of disability for children:

• requires a child to have a physical or mental condition or conditions that can be medically proven and which result in marked or severe functional limitations,

• requires that the medically proven physical or mental condition or conditions must last or be expected to last 12 months or be expected to result in death, and

• says that a child may not be considered disabled if he or she is working at a job that is considered to be substantial work.

Title XIX of the Social Security Act, **Medicaid**, is a jointly funded, federal-state program that provides health care coverage to low-income individuals and families. Medicaid eligibility is based on family size and family income. Medicaid is the largest program providing medical and health-related services to America's poorest people. Within broad national guidelines provided by the federal government, each of the states:

• establishes its own eligibility standards,

• determines the type, amount, duration, and scope of services,

• sets the rate of payment for services, and

• administers its own program.

Some of the services that children are able to receive from Medicaid include:

• inpatient hospital care, residential treatment centers, or group homes,

• clinic services by a physician or under physician direction,

• prescription drugs,

• rehabilitative services and/or outpatient hospital services,

• targeted case management, and

• when a state has obtained a waiver, home and community based services are available in place of institutional care.

EPSDT (Early and Periodic Screening, Diagnosis, and Treatment) is the child health component of the Medicaid program. Under EPSDT:

• all eligible children are entitled to periodic screening services, including comprehensive physical examinations, and vision, dental and hearing screens.

• all eligible children are entitled to any medically necessary service within the scope of the Federal program that is to correct or ameliorate defects, and physical and mental illnesses and conditions, even if the state in which the child resides has not otherwise elected to include that service in its state Medicaid plan.

Title XXI of the Social Security Act, **SCHIP (State Children's Health Insurance Program)**, is designed to provide health care for children who come from working families with incomes too high to qualify for Medicaid, but too low to afford private health insurance. Under SCHIP, the state can chose to provide child health care assistance to low-income, uninsured children through:

• a separate program,

• a Medicaid expansion, or

• a combination of these two approaches.

SCHIP targets low-income children and in most states defines them as under 19 and living in families with incomes at or below the poverty line. Children eligible for Medicaid must be enrolled in Medicaid and are not eligible for SCHIP. Also, to be eligible for SCHIP, children cannot be covered by other group health insurance. If a state chooses to expand Medicaid eligibility for its SCHIP program, the children who qualify under SCHIP are entitled to EPSDT. If a state chooses to develop a separate state program to cover children, it must include the same benefits as one of several benchmark plans (such as the state employee benefit plan, the standard Blue Cross/Blue Shield preferred provider option under the federal employee health benefit plan, or the coverage offered by an HMO with the largest commercial non-Medicaid enrollment in the state), or have an equivalent actuarial value to any one of those benchmark plans. Plans based on the equivalent actuarial value must include at least 75% of the actuarial value in the benchmark plan for mental health and substance abuse.

In administering Part B of the **Individuals with Disabilities Education Act (IDEA)**, the Office of Special Education Programs, U.S. Department of Education, helps states carry out their responsibility to provide all children with disabilities (age 3-21 years) a free appropriate public education that emphasizes special education and related services designed to meet their unique needs and prepare them for employment and independent living. Children with emotional disturbance may be eligible for special education and related services under IDEA. Additionally, some children with attention deficit hyperactivity disorder may receive services, if identified as eligible under one of the 13 specific IDEA categories of disability. Eligibility is determined by a multi-disciplinary team of qualified school professionals and parents, based on a full and individual evaluation of the child. In addition to special education delivered in the least restrictive environment, eligible children may also receive related services required to assist them benefit from special education. Examples of these services include:
- speech-language pathology and audiology services,
- psychological services,
- physical and occupational therapy,
- recreation, including therapeutic recreation,
- counseling services, including rehabilitation counseling,
- social work services in schools, and
- parent counseling and training.

Each public school child who receives special education and related services under IDEA must have an individualized education program (IEP) that details the child's goals, needed special education and services and where they will be provided, and other information. For a child whose behavior impedes his/her learning or that of others, the IEP team should consider positive behavioral interventions, strategies, and supports to address that behavior. The IDEA also provides for functional behavior assessments and development of behavioral intervention plans for students who present challenging and disruptive behaviors.

Head Start is a federal pre-school program designed to provide educational, health, nutritional, and social services, primarily in a classroom setting, to help low-income children begin school ready to learn. Head Start legislation requires that at least 90 percent of these children come from families with incomes at or below the poverty line; at least 10 percent of the enrollment slots in each local program must be available to children with disabilities. Head Start's goals include:
- developing social and learning skills, including social-emotional development,
- improving health and nutrition, and
- strengthening families' ability to provide nurturing environments through parental involvement and social services.

References for Policy Brief

Health Care Financing Administration (HCFA)
http://www.hcfa.gov/init/children.htm

Health Resources and Services Administration
(HRSA)
http://www.bphc.hrsa.gov and
http://www.hrsa.dhhs.gov/childhealth

Maternal and Child Health Bureau
http://www.mchb.hrsa.gov/index.html

Child Care Bureau
http://www.acf.dhhs.gov/programs/ccb

Insure Kids Now
http://www.insurekidsnow.gov/ and
National toll free number: 1-877-Kids-Now

Child Welfare League of America
http://www.cwla.org/health/healthfact.html

Office of Special Education Programs (OSEP)
http://www.ed.gov/offices/OSERS/OSEP

OSEP Technical Assistance Center on Positive
Behavior Interventions and Supports
http://www.pbis.org

Center for Effective Collaboration and Practice
http://cecp.air.org/cecp.html

National Center on Education, Disability, and
Juvenile Justice
http://www.edjj.org

Office of Safe and Drug-Free Schools
http://www.ed.gov/offices/OESE/SDFS

www.ingramcontent.com/pod-product-compliance
Lightning Source LLC
Chambersburg PA
CBHW081620170526
45166CB00009B/3050